D0407122

Advance praise for *The Four Desires*

"*The Four Desires* is firmly grounded in ancient wisdom. Anyone seeking inner healing and lasting happiness must read this book."
—PANDIT RAJMANI TIGUNAIT, Ph.D., chairman and spiritual head, Himalayan Institute

"*The Four Desires* is a classic of transformational writing. Accessible to anyone looking for guidance on their journey, it is one of the most helpful books I've ever read on what it requires to live a fulfilled life amid the complexities of today's world. I'm recommending it to everyone I know!"
—SALLY KEMPTON, author of *Meditation for the Love of It*

"Rod Stryker brilliantly shares countless practices to empower and satisfy your inherent longing for happiness and success, worldly as well as spiritual. *The Four Desires* is a practical, powerful guide."
—LILIAS FOLAN, PBS host and author of *Lilias! Yoga Gets Better with Age*

"*The Four Desires* is a precious gem of a book. It offers us the 'owner's manual' of time-tested teachings we all should have had available to us earlier, which we can now utilize to realize and live a life filled with purpose and meaning. I will be recommending it for years to come to all my students and teachers-in-training."
—RICHARD MILLER, Ph.D., author of *Yoga Nidra: A Meditative Practice for Deep Relaxation and Healing*

"Read *The Four Desires* slowly, savor its wisdom, and then do the exercises to help embody the wisdom. It will help you live your best life."
—ERICH SCHIFFMANN, author of *YOGA: The Spirit and Practice of Moving into Stillness*

"I am thrilled to have at my fingertips the extraordinary genius of Rod's teachings, as offered in *The Four Desires*. Regardless of one's yogic experience, Rod guides us to uncover the beauty, power, and purpose of our lives. This book is an incredible gift to have both as a teacher and student, and I am excited to use it as a resource for my own continued growth and self-discovery."
—SEANE CORN, yoga instructor and co-founder of Off the Mat, Into the World

THE
FOUR DESIRES

....

CREATING A LIFE OF PURPOSE,
HAPPINESS, PROSPERITY,
AND FREEDOM

....

ROD STRYKER

DELACORTE PRESS
NEW YORK

Published in the United States by Delacorte Press,
an imprint of The Random House Publishing Group,
a division of Random House, Inc., New York.

DELACORTE and colophon are registered
trademarks of Random House, Inc.

"Para Yoga" is a registered trademark and "The Yoga of Fulfillment"
is a trademark of Rod Stryker.

LIBRARY OF CONGRESS CATALOGING-IN-PUBLICATION DATA
Stryker, Rod.
The four desires: creating a life of purpose, happiness,
prosperity, and freedom / Rod Stryker.
p. cm.
Includes bibliographical references.
ISBN 978-0-553-80398-3 (alk. paper) 4641 9228
ISBN 978-0-440-42328-7 (eBook) 8/11
1. Yoga.   2. Success–Religious aspects–Hinduism.   I. Title.
BL1238.54.S77 2011
294.5'44—dc22   2010052828

Printed in the United States of America on acid-free paper

Illustrations by Kate Ramirez

2 4 6 8 9 7 5 3 1

FIRST EDITION

Book design by Mary A. Wirth

To my family, thank you for opening my heart wide and for the countless joys you have graced my life with.

To Jaden, Theo, Asha, and Atreya, may your paths be gentle, filled with wonder, growth, and love. May you be inspired to reach for greatness and, in so doing, add to the beauty of this world.

To my wife, Gina, you are my earth and heaven, my lover, best friend, and partner. Thank you for ever-present kindness, generosity, strength, wisdom, and enduring love.

· · · ·

CONTENTS

Afterword

. . . .

INTRODUCTION

Happiness. We all seek it. There is no more basic or universal drive than the desire to be happy. It is inherent, something we are compelled to by virtue of who and what we are.

Everything human beings have accomplished and aspired to, our every endeavor, has been and always will be rooted in the impulse to satisfy our longing for happiness. We desire love, pleasure, beauty, friendship, accomplishment, wisdom, and power. Each of us longs for an abiding sense of purpose and meaning, peace, health, and security. At some level, we also aspire to freedom, to a greater capacity to shape our destiny, and to connect with something greater than ourselves, which some call Source, Self, or God.

As the thirteenth-century poet Jalalu'ddin Rumi observed: "The wings of humankind is its aspiration." Aspiration was responsible for the creation of language, society, culture, science, architecture, the world's spiritual traditions, and even walking on the moon. Everything humanity has accomplished is the legacy of its enduring desire for fulfillment.

The book you hold in your hands is a road map to fulfilling your material and spiritual desires, both your short-term goals and the enduring longing that all human beings have, whether we're conscious of it or not, for lasting peace and freedom. The process it walks you through is based on the ancient spiritual tradition of the Vedas. A series of sacred scriptures from the land known today as India, the Vedas are, for the most part, little celebrated in the West. However, the same cannot be said for one of the Vedas' many branches—namely, yoga.

Yoga is officially an industry in America. By some estimates it generates nearly five and a half billion dollars a year. People of all walks of life, social strata, and age groups practice it: housewives, stockbrokers, professional football players, judges, country music stars, grandmothers, and schoolchildren. The reason for its widespread popularity is simple: it works.

Yoga has improved the lives of those in nursing homes in Florida, prisons in Illinois, and boardrooms in Manhattan. With research showing that children who practice yoga have higher test scores and are better adjusted socially than those who do not, some schools have begun integrating it into their curricula. Universities and hospitals nationwide are currently funding or conducting studies on yoga, as are the National Institutes of Health and the National Cancer Institute. Corporations big and small offer it to their employees. Insurance companies are underwriting yoga for their enrollees because of its proven long-term benefits: studies confirm that it slows down the aging process, reduces many stress-related symptoms, helps with back problems, and improves everything from cognitive skills to immune function to sleep, memory, and even digestion.

Despite its widespread acceptance and the number of lives it has improved, what most of us in the West commonly associate with yoga represents only the tip of the iceberg that is yoga, a tiny fraction of what is a vast and profound science; few Westerners are aware of the full breadth and power of its teachings. In fact, many people, including some who practice yoga, assume that yoga is nothing more than a form of exercise, or they believe that only the physical aspects of yoga have relevance to their lives. Nothing could be further from the truth. When yoga is understood in its totality, it is not a religion; it is a practical and comprehensive science for realizing life's ultimate aims. The yoga tradition provides one of humankind's most effective systems for achieving enrichment and happiness in every aspect of life. In short, in the same way that the physical practice of yoga so effectively benefits your body and mind, the larger science of yoga is similarly powerful in unlocking the vast potentials of your body, mind, and spirit to help you achieve your best life imaginable.

For the past three decades, I've taught yoga and meditation from this larger context of the yoga tradition. I've worked with tens of thousands *sha* is the desire to abide in deep and lasting peace, to know the Eternal; it is the aspiration to experience a boundless state, one that is beyond the reach of the other three desires.

These four desires are ever-present and fluid. In a single day you could easily experience all of them. On waking up, you might think about all your many obligations; thus your very first conscious desire might be the desire to be free from your many responsibilities, to live with no stress, and for your life to be peacefully and wholly nurturing. This desire, for ultimate freedom and freedom from worldly constraint, is *moksha*. Sooner or later you would feel hungry and desire food; if it was freezing outside, you would most likely turn on the heat. These desires for what is necessary to ensure your survival fall in the category of *artha*. It is also likely that you would want your day to be pleasurable; you might want to enjoy the company of close friends or family; you would sooner or later long to experience joy. This desire for pleasure is *kama*. Informing all of these is your soul's desire that your day, and all the days of your life, be deeply satisfying. This desire to live with purpose and meaning and to contribute to the world is *dharma*.

According to the Vedic tradition, the four desires are inherent aspects of your soul or essence; your soul uses them for the purpose of fulfilling its unique potential. Learning to honor the four desires allows you to thrive at every level and leads you to a complete and balanced life. It's important to understand that while these four desires are always present, at various times in your life, as your life's conditions change, one of the four will predominate. In other words, at any given time one of the four desires will become the most essential for you to fulfill.

The ancient tradition holds that all of us are born with an equal capacity to achieve lasting fulfillment. Desire is the seed, which can eventually lead us to it. From the viewpoint of the Vedas, all four kinds of desires, including desires for material prosperity, if pursued mindfully, can be spiritual because they can pave the way for our soul to express itself on earth. That is why an integral part of this book will provide you with a method for identifying and fulfilling those desires that are in harmony with who you are and, from your soul's perspective, who you are meant to be. Thus, *The Four Desires* and the process it leads you through are designed to enable you to uncover your life's purpose and, by helping you to cut through life's inevitable distractions, enliven your capacity to fulfill it.

Of course, not all desires lead to happiness. Desires can and do result in pain and frustration. However, according to the ancient tradition, *attachment* to desire, not desire itself, is the underlying cause of practically all of our pain and suffering. For example, attachment is the source of the pain we experience when we fail to fulfill a particular desire. It also is the source of the anxiety we feel when we do fulfill a desire but fear that we may lose what we have achieved. The yoga tradition acknowledges that the tentacles of desire—namely, attachment—can and often do lead to suffering, but the tradition also speaks at great length of the necessity of understanding your life's deeper purpose, because true happiness is dependent on your fulfilling it. Indeed, it is my observation that the failure to develop a clear understanding of their life's purpose is the reason that many people—both those who are more spiritually oriented and those who are more materially oriented—are unable to achieve and sustain the happiness that deep in their hearts they seek.

Beyond that, I also believe that many of the ills of modern society have to do with the fact that so many of us are trying to live our lives by pursuing desires that are disconnected from a greater sense of purpose and meaning. Despite all of our technological advances, practically limitless access to information, and a seemingly endless array of possibilities for short-term gratification, we live in a time when distress, mental as well as physical, is pervasive. No one is immune, neither children nor adults, neither the rich nor the poor. Indeed, the latest research shows that those of us living in affluent societies are, for the most part, no happier than those who live in far less affluent ones. Nothing, not even spiritual practice, including yoga and meditation, can make up for the failure to understand and fulfill your soul's reason for being.

Being disconnected from your life's purpose leads to pain and to any number of dysfunctional ways of coping, including abuse of alcohol, drugs, sex, and food, spending sprees, or simply living what Henry David Thoreau described as a life of "quiet desperation." On the other hand, nothing is more essential to fulfilling your inherent quest for achieving a life of lasting fulfillment than knowing your life's purpose and allowing it to guide you.

The Four Desires leads you methodically through a step-by-step process to such a life. The process that it will walk you through asks you to do more than just read about the sublime wisdom of an ancient tradition—it will ask you and show you how to apply that wisdom. The simple truth is that real fulfillment requires action. It demands that you apply skill, sensitivity, insight, courage, compassion, surrender, strength, and love. In other words, the kind of lasting fulfillment this book is designed to lead you to cannot be achieved merely by thinking about it, nor simply by making a random decision about what you want and then sitting back with an expectation that it will happen.

In my years of teaching yoga I've watched people all too often be genuinely touched and inspired by the information I will share with you, only to see them fall short in their hope of realizing life's ultimate promise for the simple reason that they failed to apply what they had learned. Their experience is an invaluable lesson if we choose to acknowledge it: in matters of spirit as well as everyday life, without skillfully applying your knowledge, you will rarely be able to change yourself or your life for the better, nor will you be able to fulfill your deepest aspirations. An ancient text, the *Mahanirvana Tantra,* says it succinctly: *siddhi* (a Sanskrit term that means "accomplishment, achievement, or success") is produced by *sadhana* (a Sanskrit term meaning "practice"). In other words, success is less the result of what you *know* than the cumulative effect of what you *do.*

As you will soon see, I have written *The Four Desires* to be a personal and interactive process. The book is meant to function like a course in which I walk you through a series of steps to follow, exactly as if you were participating in a live seminar. I developed and began teaching just such a course more than a decade ago. I continue to teach it today. I call it the Yoga of Fulfillment. Seeing the process change thousands of lives for the better inspired me to adapt it into the book you are reading.

Throughout this book you will find key teachings, drawn from the ancient tradition, that detail how to achieve a fulfilled life—in both worldly and spiritual terms. You will also find exercises and techniques that will allow you to apply these teachings in order for you to realize your unique version of fulfillment. Along with these teachings and exercises, I have included real-life stories of people (with names changed to protect privacy) who have done the process—both those who achieved their desires and those who did not.

Part I of *The Four Desires* provides the philosophical groundwork of the process and is dedicated to helping you understand, from the point of view of the ancient teachings, the nature of desire and your own desires and how to see them in light of your soul's purpose.

Part II will walk you through the process of uncovering your soul's unique purpose and thereby establish a life strategy, which will provide the basis to chart your course for long-term happiness and fulfillment. In addition to giving you a foundation for a life of real meaning and purpose, having this kind of life strategy will also provide you with a frame of reference to know exactly which one of your many desires is the most important for you to respond to at any given time.

Then Part III will help you determine the specific desire that your soul aspires to achieve now. The process you will use to pinpoint this specific desire is one that you will be able to use time and time again to identify and achieve the goals to which you truly aspire.

Part IV takes you through several steps that will significantly increase your capacity to fulfill your desires. Parts V and VI walk you through the principles of how to live with more joy. They will explore the key principles of the yoga tradition's approach to lasting happiness and detail how to continue to apply the principles of *The Four Desires* long after you've finished reading the book.

You Can Do Yoga and Not Do Postures

I close each of the six parts of the book with a brief description of a single yoga pose (*asana*) and a commentary on how that particular posture relates to the subject of the part. I believe these commentaries will be of value to you even if you've never done yoga postures and never intend to do them.

The practice of *asana* invites us to embody all of life's greatest and most enduring qualities, including courage, willpower, self-awareness, concentration, surrender or letting go, the pursuit of excellence, the empowerment that comes from overcoming resistance (both internal and external), and skillful action.

Each of the six parts of this book is dedicated to discussing at least one of these themes. Each part ends with an illustration of one pose that seems to me to embody the theme we have been exploring. By shedding light on the ways in which certain qualities of the pose connect to the subject matter, I hope to show you how simply reflecting on the posture, even if you've never done it, can help you gain access to another level of insight. If you have done yoga *asanas*, this will give you a way to view the experience of your practice within the larger scope of your life. For those who haven't done *asanas*, these reflections on the poses might be of interest because they shed light on how the physical practice of yoga is more than just physical. In either case, these commentaries are not intended to be instructions for doing the pose; they are intended to support the larger intent of the book—to lead you to honor the most sacred part of yourself by living your best life possible.

The Power of Mind

Each part of the book features a different meditation practice. I've included these practices to help you gain insight into the process of achieving material and spiritual fulfillment. One reason that meditation has been a part of practically every spiritual tradition since time immemorial is that it provides so many benefits: physical, mental, and emotional, as well as spiritual. What's more, contrary to what many people think, meditation does not have to be complicated—or to have a religious affiliation—to be highly effective. Simply put, meditation is the process of learning to focus your mind and eventually to rest in greater levels of stillness and peace, which is why it helps anyone and everyone who will practice it.

Even if you have never meditated before, you will find the meditations that I have included inspiring, yet accessible. If you follow the step-by-step instructions that I have carefully laid out, I am certain you will discover that each of these meditations has the potential to benefit you in countless ways.

How to Use This Book

I've said that in order to get the maximum benefit from *The Four Desires,* you will need to do the exercises, which have been organized systematically. However, you do not necessarily have to do the exercises the first time you read the book. You may find yourself wanting to read everything that leads up to and follows the exercises and skip doing them the first time through. If that's the case, as you read the principles for achieving your goals and the stories that show how people have applied—or failed to apply—these principles for fulfillment, focus on how they touch you and relate to your life and what you truly desire. Then, drawing upon what you've read as inspiration and motivation, return to the exercises and do them in the order prescribed.

Some of the exercises will require relatively little work on your part and will take only a few minutes. Others, particularly in Parts II and III, are more involved and require more time and thought. Whichever way you prefer to approach the material, the important thing is that you eventually apply the systematic steps and exercises that I've laid out.

I believe you will find—as have most of the people whose stories I tell in these pages—that once you have worked with the process in *The Four Desires*, you will want to use the exercises and methods as a regular part of your life. The practices of identifying your soul's desires and applying ancient, time-tested methodology to effectively fulfill them are remarkably powerful in leading you to a life of greater purpose, happiness, prosperity, and lasting freedom. Therefore, I designed *The Four Desires* as a process to be used over and over.

The Journey to Eternal Fulfillment

Obviously, desire and achieving fulfillment have their challenges. First, there is the challenge of knowing what you want—which for some of us is less than clear. Second, there is the challenge of trying to decipher whether or not what you want is really in your best interests: is it coming from your "higher self" or from some less desirable place? The third challenge is getting what you want. Fourth is the issue of how to live with the expectations or attachments that invariably accompany our desires and which the ancient tradition makes clear are the root of the majority of our suffering. And finally, there's the challenge of finding meaning and satisfaction throughout the course of your life whether or not you attain your specific desires.

The Four Desires addresses each of these challenges and shows you how to successfully navigate them. Along the way, it will teach you how to build your energy and direct your resolve to fulfill your life's highest calling. The process through which I will lead you has been refined over many years. I am confident that if you apply it, your life will be improved in countless ways. Nonetheless, as much as I value, trust, and believe in the process, I offer it to you in the same spirit as the teachings of the Upanishads, ancient texts that provide some of the most elevated teachings of yogic science. The Upanishads tell the reader, "Follow that advice of mine which is good and helpful for your progress, and neglect even my own advice which is not."

I wish to acknowledge the endless succession of luminous teachers who, from time immemorial, have lit a golden path to eternal fulfillment and chosen to leave us the legacy of their experiences—a science of true auspiciousness, the highest kind of success and happiness. That timeless journey is what this book is all about. It is dedicated to helping you learn to hear destiny's call and to answer it with your best life. The chapters that lie ahead map the journey to fulfill life's ultimate promise, the one all human beings long for and that is hailed in one of India's most revered texts, the *Srimad Bhagavatam*: "Deep within lies a real and everlasting joy. A human being is born to dive deep into the stream of life, find the hidden treasure, and attain eternal fulfillment."

Eternal fulfillment is both an art and a science. By learning to skill-fully apply the science, you become an artist, whereby your heart's deepest desires become your brushstrokes and your finished canvas becomes the life you were meant to share with the world. Join me now as you begin the journey of *The Four Desires*.

PART I

. . . .

LIFE IS DESIRE

CHAPTER 1

. . . .

THE POWER OF DESIRE

Ten years before I met Dean, he was at the top of his career as a broadcast journalist. After more than a decade covering a variety of conflicts in the Middle East and Asia, he was now appearing nightly on network television. Just when it seemed that he had attained everything he had ever aspired to and spent his life working for, Dean's life as he knew it came to a devastating end. He had experienced various levels of excruciating pain for the past six years after suffering a fractured vertebra and declining surgery. But now he knew that something was terribly wrong. Rushed into emergency surgery, he woke from general anesthesia to a doctor standing over him, giving him the grave news that the operation had "failed" and that Dean would be "permanently disabled."

Unable to sit, barely able to walk, Dean returned to the States, literally and figuratively a broken man, his spirit as broken as his spine, his career over. Within months, he was little more than what he described as a man "pickled on painkillers."

Over the next couple of years, little changed—until his wife gave birth to their first child. His time celebrating Finn's birth was cut short, however. Dean's health, which had been deteriorating since the failed surgery, had taken a turn for the worse. Tests revealed a new, life-altering diagnosis: cancer. His prognosis was "a year or two to live." With his physical pain and mental torment more severe than ever, Dean's doses of prescription painkillers were increased and now included a morphine drip.

Months passed with Dean bedridden and in all but a hopeless state. Then, with less than a year to live, Dean had an epiphany. Lying in bed with his young son playing nearby, the nightmare of the past few years and the weight of dying suddenly came crushing down on him. He was overwhelmed by the realization that he was moving irreversibly toward fulfilling the doctors' prognosis; he and his son—the most precious thing in the world to him—would soon be separated forever.

Suddenly, as though breaking through the dark cloud that had been overshadowing his whole life the past few years, Dean saw himself through the eyes of his son. If nothing changed and he was to die, Finn's only memory of his father would be that of a man who had *committed* to nothing other than being a helpless victim. Dean realized that he had so succumbed to self-pity that his son had never seen his father do or be anything that Finn could look back on and be proud of. It was not Dean's fault that he broke his back or had cancer, but Finn had not seen him even try to make the best of the time he did have—that was Dean's responsibility. Someone somewhere in the world had it worse than he did, Dean realized, and someone somewhere was doing better than he was with far less.

Dean immediately made a resolution. He would change. There was no way to know if he would survive cancer or ever be an able-bodied father who could play baseball with his son, but he made a commitment nonetheless. For however many days he had left, he would be a living example to his son of how a man could, or in Dean's eyes should, live his life. He would face the circumstances in his life exactly as he would want Finn to face his own future challenges.

A few days later, Dean found himself doing yoga for the first time in a class that was being offered at his rehabilitation center. Within minutes, he knew he had, in his words, "found his path to healing." He had no way of knowing whether the healing would be spiritual and physical or just spiritual, but he sensed that it was the beginning of a new chapter in his life.

Driven by his resolve, Dean immersed himself in learning everything he could about well-being, spirituality, and cancer therapies and applying what he learned. He consumed books on diet and nutrition, yoga, spirituality, positive thinking, visualization, and meditation. He dramatically changed his lifestyle, inside and out. He willed himself to practice yoga and meditation for hours a day—in the beginning, crawling out of bed to get onto his yoga mat.

As the months passed, things began to change. Dean could sit up for ten, then twenty, then eventually sixty minutes at a time. Soon after that, he was able to walk to the kitchen. He cut back on his pain medication and eventually stopped it altogether. More victories came. Eventually he was able to drive. And then came the one change that meant more to him than any of the others: he was able to lift and hold his son. Miraculously, and to his doctors' amazement, Dean had healed his broken back. But his transformation didn't end there. A short time later, about the time he was supposed to be dead, Dean received a new diagnosis: he was "cancer-free."

> . . . .
>
> *"The important thing is this: to be able, at any moment, to sacrifice what we are for what we could become."*
>
> —CHARLES DU BOS
>
> . . . .

Dean's story is extraordinary. A person can do all that he did (and more) and still not be cured of cancer or heal a broken back, but his is more than a story about beating the odds. It is an illustration of the *power of desire* coupled with the willingness to use every resource available to achieve a goal. It is a telling reminder of just how potent you can be in affecting your destiny. Viewed from a different perspective, Dean's story can also be seen as ordinary, in the sense that it portrays the very definition of what constitutes a human being, what in Sanskrit is called a *kama yoni,* which means "the species which has the privilege of performing actions and which thus can change the course of its destiny." By seizing his resolve and taking positive command of all the resources available to him, Dean was embodying the principle that defines us and sets us apart from all other species.

This idea was eloquently expressed by French essayist Charles Du Bos, who I believe conveyed the essence of all yogic teachings as well as the formula for achieving a truly fulfilled life when he wrote, "The important thing is this: to be able, at any moment, to sacrifice what we are for what we could become."

Take a moment to consider who you would be and how much better our world would be if more of us would "sacrifice what we are for what we could become."

Dean came to one of my Yoga of Fulfillment workshops after he had healed physically. Wanting a clearer understanding of what had transformed him, he was hoping to make use of the same power to overcome the current challenges in his life. Working with the processes of the Yoga of Fulfillment allowed Dean to see that having to face the prospect of imminent death, of being permanently separated from his son, had been the catalyst he needed to be willing to change his life. His intention to be "a living example" to his son for whatever time he had left altered the course of his destiny.

Dean's miracle-like accomplishments had everything to do with his willingness to sacrifice what he *was* in order to become what he *could* be. It began by him acknowledging his desire and finding a specific goal that he knew deep in his heart was absolutely worth achieving. Dean's overriding desire was to give his son a father he could love, respect, and perhaps even one day emulate. The Yoga of Fulfillment helped him realize that he had intuitively applied the principles that the ancient tradition teaches are key to achieving our goals. Once he learned the principles, he was able to apply them systematically to successfully meet the new challenges in his life.

Dean's intuitive unearthing of a singular and compelling purpose for his life combined with his all-consuming commitment to fulfilling it is a powerful illustration of a profound truth that was something of a credo for my first teacher, Mani. Drawing from an ancient scripture, he would constantly repeat, "A person can achieve almost anything, can surmount any difficulties, if they can harness their power."

The good news is that you don't need to be facing life-and-death circumstances, as Dean was, to harness this power. As Mani reminded me time and time again, you have extraordinary power to accomplish extraordinary things—enough to "achieve almost anything" and "surmount any difficulties"—if you are willing to formulate goals and learn how to direct your innate power toward achieving them. The foundation for achieving any and all that you aspire to is the power of desire.

Desire Is Everything and Everywhere

Desire touches everything in the natural world. It is easy to lose sight of just how powerful, pervasive, and integral desire is to the world in which you and I live. If not for a spark between your biological father's sperm and biological mother's egg, you wouldn't exist. Thanks to one particularly desirous sperm, you are in your present form, reading these words. Congratulations. You are, in fact, the winner of an intense competition between millions of other microscopic sperm desirous of impregnating an egg.

At your birth, more than your mother's desire was necessary to bring you into the world. If you were born naturally, *you* actively engaged in a most intense sequence of what are unmistakably willful and desirous contortions to pass through your mother's birth canal. And just in case the sum of your and your mother's desires had not been enough to bring you into the world safely, it would have been necessary to rely on the desire of doctors and other caregivers to intervene. "Man is verily formed of desire," the *Brihadaranyaka Upanishad* reminds us.

Desire's role didn't end when you came into the world. Desire compelled you to lift your head and then to roll over and later to stand; once you were able to stand, desire compelled you to walk, then to run. Thanks to desire, you sought to develop the skill of language, in large part so you could more clearly ask for—if not insist on—the things you *wanted* as well as to participate with those around you. Speaking, and later writing, provided you more freedom and capacity to pursue your desires in life. You are who and what you are *because* of desire.

God of the Old Testament had desires. His desires were the first sparks that created light and life, day and night, heaven and earth, and the stars. Before any of them existed, according to the Judeo-Christian tradition, each was a flicker of desire in the eye of the Almighty. The same concept is found in the spiritual traditions of India. The *Yajur Veda*, for example, one of the four original Vedic texts, tells us that divine desire, or *kama*, created the world. Without this desire, the world could not exist.

The Vedas teach that desire is ever-present. It is with you at every step and with every breath you take. Desire precedes your every action, since before you can *do*, you first have to *want*. I can't lift my arm, reach for a drink of water, or do anything else without first wanting to; thus every action you have done or will do—including those that are sparked by your subconscious—is preceded by a desire.

Desire is also the seed of every thought. The tradition teaches that before you can have a thought, you first have to have a desire. Imagine how many thoughts you have had in your lifetime and you'll begin to have an idea how many desires you have had.

"As long as one has a body, one cannot renounce action altogether," says the Bhagavad Gita. Thus, for all practical purposes, as long as you are acting, thinking, or speaking—as long as you are alive—there is no end to desire.

Desire, the same thing that possessed the part of you that at one time was the sperm to fertilize the other part of you that was the egg, is the same thing that compels your lungs to breathe, your heart to beat, your kidneys to function, your body, in all its complexity, to work as an integrated whole. This same spark also fuels your desire for spiritual and lasting fulfillment and motivates you to seek fulfillment in every facet of life.

To paraphrase T. K. V. Desikachar, a renowned author and widely considered a leading voice for the ancient tradition of yoga, the first step in yoga is the *desire* to be better. Alain Daniélou, a highly respected authority on Vedic wisdom, in his book *Virtue, Success, Pleasure, and Liberation,* cites Madhavacharya: "On the physical, as on the intellectual and spiritual plane, all creation, all invention, all imagination is the fruit of desire."

Even the Buddha, who, it is fair to say, transcended desire, preached what he called the Middle Way or Middle Path, which is the path, according to the Buddha, that led to the state of enlightenment. He described it as the balance between the extremes of sensual indulgence and total renunciation. It is also worth noting that a deep and profound aspiration was what moved the Buddha to pursue and eventually achieve enlightenment. In other words, without a highly evolved desire to overcome suffering and the pain of impermanence, he would not have achieved sublime exaltation; he would not have been moved to search for a way to end his own suffering and then, after he achieved it, to alleviate it in those he saw around him.

Desire is here to stay. The challenge we all face, and which I intend to guide you through, is to learn how to take into account the full measure of who you are and use the positive force of all four of your soul's desires—*dharma,* the desire to become who you were meant to be; *artha,* the desire for the means to help you fulfill your *dharma; kama,* the desire for pleasure of all kinds; and *moksha,* the desire for freedom and a connection to the Eternal—to lead you to your best life.

CHAPTER 2

. . . .

TWO KINDS OF FULFILLMENT

The Oxford American Dictionary defines *fulfillment* as "satisfaction or happiness as a result of fully developing one's abilities or character," and as "the achievement of something desired, promised, or predicted." It's worth noting that both aspects of this definition are attainment-oriented, something you feel whenever you satisfy a want or desire, or reach a goal.

You first experienced this kind of fulfillment early in life when, for example, you were provided with milk in response to your cries. This kind of fulfillment continued, evolving into the elation you probably felt on Christmas morning if the presents you hoped for were under the tree, the pride of receiving the merit badge you aspired to as a Boy or Girl Scout, the pleasure of buying something you really wanted, the excitement of your first kiss or your first sexual experience, the high of a promotion at work, the thrill of your stocks going up, the joy of discovering that someone you are attracted to feels the same way about you. The more you've desired something, the longer you've waited for it, the more of this kind of fulfillment you are likely to experience when it's finally yours. At least for a while.

The pull to find happiness through this kind of fulfillment is a powerful and commanding force. The life of almost every human being— every one of us except perhaps a true saint or sage—is entirely influenced by it. Though the specifics of what will provide you with this kind of fulfillment will surely change over the course of your life, the longing to achieve it will not. It endures to the instant before your last breath—when the object of your desire will likely be another lifetime of breaths. Fulfillment through attainment—whether the object be material or nonmaterial, substantial like a car or intangible like a particular emotion you long to feel—is preeminent, and perhaps that is why it is the only definition you find in the dictionary.

There is another kind of fulfillment that the dictionary fails to include—a kind, most spiritual traditions assert, that is critical to understand and ultimately learn to embody if you are going to realize true or lasting happiness and fulfillment. This other type of fulfillment is not dependent on attainment or on any thing. It is based on a recognition, a shift in perception. You could even say it is a revelation. The second kind of fulfillment is not dependent on circumstances being just right, nor is it derived from anything in the outside world. It comes from you. It *is* you. "It is not inaccessible nor is it in distant places: it is what in oneself appears to be the experience of bliss, and is therefore realized in oneself." This quote from the *Yoga Vasistha,* one of the most comprehensive and esteemed yogic scriptures, reveals everything you need to know about the kind of fulfillment not mentioned in the dictionary. This kind of fulfillment is usually hidden, masked by the world of things—the world that most of us normally see and with which we engage.

This other fulfillment is constantly and permanently available, provided you know how to access silence. "Only by the stilled mind can he be known," says the *Shvetashvatara Upanishad;* or as Psalms 46:10 of the King James Bible tells us, "Be still and know that I am God." In other words, only when you find a way to still the otherwise endless pursuit for the first kind of fulfillment can and will you be able to realize the second kind.

Fulfillment of this kind doesn't wait for your dream lover to appear, for a breakthrough in your career, for the roses to start blooming in your garden, or for your child to finally come home with good grades. Fulfillment of this kind is always available because it emanates from something that is unchanging. It is, therefore, a complete and enduring fulfillment. It is, as we are informed by every spiritual tradition, a kind of wealth far beyond the riches and accomplishments found in the material world. It is an indestructible treasure, one that can never be lost or taken away. Throughout the ages, it has been described in various ways as the unfolding of the most glorious presence, a contentment that words can never fully convey.

As lofty as this second type of fulfillment might sound, it is important to understand that you do not have to choose one or the other; indeed, for most of us, both are crucial to leading a rich and fulfilled life. However, not everyone, and certainly not every spiritual tradition, sees it that way. It is not uncommon that some of us, consciously or unconsciously, believe that we have to choose one kind of fulfillment over the other. In my experience, the people most prone to believing that they have to make a choice between one or the other are those seeking "spiritual" fulfillment. Unfortunately, I've seen how this kind of either/or point of view can have a negative impact on people on both sides of the material-versus-spiritual debate, making it harder to achieve any kind of genuine fulfillment.

As my teacher Pandit Rajmani Tigunait explains in his book *Tantra Unveiled*:

> According to most spiritual traditions the desire for worldly pleasure is incompatible with the spiritual quest. You can have the treasures of this world, they say, or the treasures of the spiritual realm, but not both. This either/or approach sets off an endless internal struggle in those who are drawn to spiritual beliefs and practices but who have at the same time a natural urge to fulfill their worldly desires. This includes most of us. And when there is no way to reconcile these two impulses we fall prey to guilt and self-condemnation, or we repress either our spiritual desires or our worldly desires, or we try to have both, and become hypocrites.

The Best of Both Worlds

The very first time I did yoga, I discovered a greater sense of peace than I had ever known. Each subsequent time I did it, I can honestly say it led me to feel inspired, more capable, and clearer about myself and the world. But when I first started studying the teachings of yoga, I couldn't help noticing a contradiction between the way yoga practice made me feel and what I understood at the time about its teachings, which seemed rather unforgiving when it came to desires—even the most basic emotional and biological ones. Unless you practiced celibacy, for instance, it seemed you would wind up as just another lost soul. I inferred that I could also toss my creative impulses and worldly ambitions into the same heap with everything else in my life that was in conflict with yoga's aim to transcend the highs and lows of living in the material world.

It was confusing to feel drawn to the promise of physical, mental, and spiritual enrichment that my experiences in yoga were providing me with, while knowing that I desired a family, a vital creative life, a way to express my talents and capacities, and of course the money to take care of myself and my future family. My conflict helps to explain why I practiced yoga so intensely but sporadically for the first couple of years. For spiritual fulfillment, would I have to forgo all worldly desires, goals, and pleasures? To pursue and attain worldly fulfillment, would I need to forgo yoga?

The answer to both questions, I would later discover, was no. But at the time, I didn't know this. Based on the little I had read and the common assumptions that I held, I didn't know that yoga could embrace both material and worldly fulfillment. That's because my initial exposure to yoga philosophy and teachings appeared only to stress the path of renunciation, what the Vedic tradition refers to as *nivritti marga*. *Marga* means "path"; *nivritti* means "completion or termination." Its overriding intention is *moksha* or liberation. Its underlying philosophy is that only through renunciation of the world and all desire can one achieve ultimate freedom and find *the* path to true and lasting happiness.

About the time I concluded that the yoga tradition held little promise in helping me achieve the life I truly aspired to, I met Mani, my first teacher. He made it clear that *nivritti*—complete denial of our senses, our individuality, and our desire—was all but impossible; it was mostly a theoretical concept that could be applied by only the rarest of individuals. An ancient scripture, the *Mahanirvana Tantra,* makes it very clear: "The thirst for life will continue to manifest itself until the point of return is reached and the outgoing energy is exhausted. Man must, until such time, remain on the path of desire. . . . One cannot renounce until one has enjoyed." According to Vedic wisdom, the path of *nivritti* is not an appropriate path for those with obligations such as family, work still to do in this world, or enduring desires yet to be fulfilled.

Mani laid out another vision of yoga that was suited to those of us who have desires and goals in the material world as well as spiritual desires. The path that is appropriate for most of us is called *pravritti marga.* The path of *pravritti* is the path of expansion, moving outward and toward accomplishment. Instead of transcending all desires, this path uses the fuel of desire to lead us to happiness. As does the path of *nivritti,* it includes the idea that your Source is limitless and eternal—a wellspring of boundless vitality, wisdom, and love—but instead of seeing this Essence as separate from this world, it perceives its beauty as a seamless expression of it.

The path of *pravritti* teaches that the objects of the world are outward expressions of the Divine. As the Upanishads say, "All—whatsoever that moves in the universe—is indwelt by the Lord. . . . Enjoy thou what hath been allotted by Him." Desire, instead of being an obstacle to an inspired and fulfilled life, is the very thing that propels you toward it. "Desire is the essence of all action," says the *Mahabharata,* the world's longest epic poem (of which the highly revered Bhagavad Gita is a part). In fact, we find in the Gita, "Both renunciation of action and the selfless performance of action lead to the supreme goal. But the path of action is better than renunciation." Striving and activity are part of life, so *pravritti* teaches you to see the world—with all its challenges, ups and downs, and apparent flaws—as the ideal place to fully realize your spiritual potential as well as to enjoy all that life has to offer.

> . . . .
>
> *Desire, instead of being an obstacle to an inspired and fulfilled life, is the very thing that propels you toward it.*
>
> . . . .

To live in the world in a way that can yield the treasure of deep and lasting fulfillment does not require you to deny or suppress desire. Instead, the tradition instructs, you need to learn to temper your desires with discretion to ensure that they are a vibrant expression of your best self and will therefore lead you to real and lasting satisfaction. "Desire is not to be let loose without bridle," the *Mahanirvana Tantra,* another revered thirteenth-century text, tells us. The bridle, as I'll show you throughout the book, is the guidance of your Source or soul, the ever-present source of wisdom and compassion that you can learn to tap into.

Nivritti and *pravritti* are the two paths that the ancient tradition prescribes for reaching life's ultimate goal. They share the same intention: to provide a means to find and attain supreme happiness. What primarily sets these two paths apart is how they relate to desire. One path requires suppression or elimination of all worldly desires. The other focuses on learning how to most adeptly express desire or heavenly inspiration, Spirit, or Essence in the world.

Most Eastern spiritual traditions, and certainly the Vedas, teach that these two paths need not be separate. They teach that learning to know your highest Self can coexist with an embrace of the world, family, friends, creativity, the beauty of Nature, the warmth and pleasures of love—and even the occasional hot fudge sundae. The place where the best of these two paths converge is the destination that *The Four Desires* is dedicated to helping you reach. It is also the basis of the approach to living an extraordinary life that Mani first introduced me to: the ancient tradition of tantra.

Tantra: Weaving the Threads of Material and Spiritual Prosperity

What is tantra? Tantra acknowledges and incorporates the material and spiritual in its concept of the universe. It affirms what the Vedas tell us about the inseparability of the material world from our existence as human beings, and teaches that no desire is inherently good or bad. My teacher Panditji summed it up beautifully: "Tantra is the way to discover the infinite potential of your body, the power of your mind, and the beauty of your soul." In short, tantra is dedicated to helping you prosper in every area of your life.

The word *tantra* has many meanings; each helps shed some light and understanding on what is an incomparably vast and profound spiritual tradition.

Tantra is the compound of two Sanskrit words, *tan,* which means "to expand or stretch," and *tra,* which means "that which protects." *Tantra* literally means "that which allows us to safely expand or grow beyond all limitation." An essential premise of tantra is that we are all under the influence of certain limitations. These limitations can refer to any of the following: our limited perception, our conditioning, our finances, our beliefs, the influence of the stars (astrological), our diet, our energetic state, or our environmental (social or cultural) limitations, to name just a few. The practices you employ to overcome these and any other limitations are, by definition, *tantric.*

One of the most ancient meanings of the word *tantra* is "to weave."

In this sense, *tantra* refers to the philosophy and techniques that allow us to weave the richness of spiritual experience and the fabric of everyday life into a single vibrant tapestry. Dissolving the apparent conflict between the spiritual (the Infinite) and the worldly (the finite) and thereby achieving both kinds of fulfillment, is the heart of tantric philosophy and practice.

Tantric philosophy sees the world and everything in it as a manifestation of Sri, the most radiant and resplendent aspect of the Divine. Tantric seers viewed the material world and the skillful use of all the objects in it as potential means to achieve the full flowering of spiritual experience, where the Infinite and the finite could be exalted simultaneously. They viewed the physical world, the world in which you and I live, as heaven. "What is here is elsewhere; what is not here is nowhere," says the *Mahanirvana Tantra*.

Tantric visionaries stressed that it is neither helpful nor necessary to delay seeking heaven until the afterlife. However, according to tantra, while you are still living in the world and occupying a physical body, you can only realize heaven if you awaken your dormant potential. To do that, it is necessary to employ the right methodology. Practitioners of tantra developed systematic approaches, working with everything available to them, including their physical bodies, breath, senses, mind, diet, alchemy, astrology, architecture, geometry, visualization, the power of intention, deep relaxation, mantra, and, of course, yoga. All of these practices, including the tantric approach to yoga, are for the purpose of awakening otherwise hidden powers or capacities. As my teacher Pandit Rajmani Tigunait explains:

> Tantric masters discovered long ago that success in both the outer world and the spiritual realm is possible only if we awaken our latent power, because any meaningful accomplishment, and especially the attainment of the ultimate spiritual goal, requires great strength and stamina. The key to success is *shakti*—the power of soul, the power of the divine force within. Everyone possesses an infinite (and indomitable) *shakti*, but for the most part it remains dormant. And those whose *shakti* is largely unawakened have neither the capacity to be successful in the world nor the capacity to enjoy worldly pleasures. Without access to our *shakti*, true spiritual illumination is not possible. Awakening and using *shakti* is the goal of tantra.

The point of this teaching is that the more you are able to access *shakti,* the power of soul, the more capable you are of achieving whatever goal you are seeking. The various techniques and approaches throughout this book, all adapted from tantric wisdom, are to help you harness your soul's power and to ensure that you express all of its wondrous capacities in your life.

Stories abound of tantric masters who, having mastered this power, have been able to manifest miracle-like occurrences such as—believe it or not—materializing objects out of thin air, affecting the future, being able to bilocate (be in two places at once), and even bringing the dead back to life. Authoritative tantric practitioners do not view as ends in themselves the extraordinary capacities to transcend natural law that some masters have reputedly shown. Rather, they view these capacities as a demonstration of the potential power that all human beings have to generate more auspiciousness—to attract more happiness and success at every level.

> . . . .
>
> *The more you are able to access* shakti, *the power of soul, the more capable you are of achieving whatever goal you are seeking.*
>
> . . . .

Although the power of tantric practice to affect material change makes it particularly relevant for those of us searching for ways to more effectively achieve fulfillment, it is also true that human beings' fascination with spectacular feats has helped contribute to some of the widespread confusion about tantra. In many parts of India today, for instance, tantra is known less for the profound spiritual tradition that it actually is and more as a form of magic. The West has seen a different distortion and misinterpretation of tantra. In recent decades, a handful of Westerners began teaching exotic sexual practices and identifying them as "tantric." As a result, until a few years ago most people in the West who knew of tantra most likely associated it with a marathon-like approach to "spiritual sex." Without a doubt, there has been a share of both Western and Eastern charlatans throughout the ages who called their distorted teachings tantra, which has led to a great deal of misinformation.

Another reason for the confusion that has often surrounded tantra has to do with the sheer diversity of its subject matter. Depending on which of its many aspects you focus on, you could easily conclude that it is exclusively materialistic, ritualistic, sensual, profane, superstitious, psychological, supernatural, spiritual, devotional, arcane, epistemological, or simply magical. None of this applies to the way we'll use the teachings. Our focus will be practical and straightforward: to help you have more of what you want and less of what you don't want, while at the same time honoring all of who you are.

One of the most important meanings of the word *tantra* is "system," "method," or "technique." In the same way you use technology throughout your day to start your car, boil an egg, set your alarm clock, and so on, tantric science and the methods developed from it can help make your life more efficient and effective, can help give you more freedom. Tantra, therefore, is the application of any technique or system that moves you beyond your limitations and closer to the objects and the life you seek.

I'll close with what is perhaps the least-known meaning of the word *tantra,* which is "to be touched," referring specifically to the concept of your heart being touched. Think of the last time you felt a sense of awe, wonder, or profound appreciation for life, when you suddenly saw life as the greatest of all gifts. That moment might have happened when you were alone or on a crowded city street, looking into the eyes of your child, hearing the national anthem, or tossing a Frisbee to your dog. At that moment, you recognized that while life may be complicated, unpredictable, and full of challenges, you are nonetheless blessed to be alive.

That moment, when all sense of limitation fell away, is tantra. The vast array of techniques, practices, and teachings that tantric masters developed through the centuries are for the purpose of awakening you to this experience, and enabling you to weave it more and more consistently into the tapestry of your life. And that is also the goal of all the processes in this book, which are either drawn directly from or inspired by tantric wisdom.

CHAPTER 3

. . . .

THE FOUR DESIRES

For the Purpose of Soul

A human being is meant to do more and achieve more than just survive. We all seek material security and happiness, but our spirit, soul, or essence longs for something greater than what temporal pleasure and mere survival can provide.

The concept of desire coming from the soul or essence may seem strange since, by definition, the soul is eternal and changeless. But the Vedas explain that the soul has two aspects: it is complete, whole, and eternal, in a permanent state of oneness with the Absolute, and at the same time, it desires to fully express itself and its divine nature in the world. The Vedic term for "soul" is *atman,* which means "essence," the highest principle, or Self. The two distinct aspects of *atman* are *para* and *jiva*. *Para* means "supreme, highest, or culmination." *Jiva* means "individual or personal."

The *paramatman* or higher soul is the infinite and unconditioned essence that is beyond all limitation, eternal and changeless. The *Shve-tashvatara Upanishad,* a sacred text from the seventh century, describes this higher aspect of soul beautifully: "Omnipresent, dwelling in the heart of every living creature . . . He is the inner Self of all, hidden like a little flame in the heart. . . . Know Him and all fetters will fall away." The Apostle Paul, in Corinthians 3:16, points to this same aspect of soul: "Know ye not that ye are the temple of God and that the Spirit of God dwelleth in you?" Your *paramatman* is identical to the Divine; there is no separation or distinction. "*Ahum brahma smi*" (I am one with the Absolute), say the Vedas.

Jivatman, on the other hand, is the individual soul. Think of it as your spiritual thumbprint, utterly unique for everyone. It is the part of you that, from the moment you were conceived, determines your uniqueness, your distinct capacities, talents, and challenges as well as your inclinations and desires. *Jivatman* is literally where your soul meets your unconscious—the individual aspects of you that make you uniquely who you are.

I first became familiar with the Vedic teaching about the nature of soul many years ago, but it was not until my twin sons were born that I had practical proof of its accuracy, for I saw from the very beginning of their lives how the concept of *jivatman* applied to them. My boys Jaden and Theo were conceived at the same time and gestated in the same womb, where they consumed the same nutrients. They were born only ten minutes apart, yet from the moment they came into the world they have been utterly distinct. Theo, for example, was born with an incredible ear for music. Days after he was born, we noticed that music would completely captivate him. Jaden, on the other hand, showed little response to music; he came into the world with much more tactile awareness. A gentle rub on his back and he would be spellbound. I can also recall him, at just a couple of months old, clenching my shirt and trying to climb upward. A few months later he could work his way up to the top of my head. Ten years later he's still a relentless climber. Theo has turned out to have a pitch-perfect ear and is now an inspired pianist. Now that they are in the world, their environment will undoubtedly affect their inherent qualities in a variety of ways, but what made them, from the beginning of their lives, who they are and who they will potentially become is their *jivatman,* their individual souls.

The ancient wisdom of the Vedas teaches that each of us is both universal and unique, that the two aspects of the soul, *para* and *jiva,* are distinct but not separate. The nature of the *paramatman* is that it is identical to Infinite Being. *Jiva* or individual soul, on the other hand, comes into the world with a specific purpose, which it is compelled to fulfill. In the same way that there are specific genetic traits in a tulip bulb that will determine its color, the shape of its petals, and the time it will most likely bloom, the *jiva* of Wolfgang Amadeus Mozart, Leonardo da Vinci, and

Albert Einstein contained the unique potentialities of their destiny the moment they were conceived.

Dharma

As I described in the introduction, your soul, specifically the *jiva* aspect of your soul, has four desires that it uses to propel you toward your unique destiny. The first and most overriding of the four desires is *dharma*, the longing for purpose, the drive to be and to become who you are meant to be. *Dharma*, in simple terms, is the drive to fulfill your potential; it is the inherent drive of every being to thrive. *Dharma* is also the impulse toward altruism, the inner longing, known or unknown, of every individual to add his or her unique luster to the gem of creation. The term *dharma* has many meanings, including "law," "path," "order," and "virtue." Each of these definitions helps to define *dharma* as *the* one desire that informs the other three desires. In the yoga tradition, *dharma* is often referred to as duty. *Dharma*, in the context of the four desires, is usually interpreted to mean career, life path, or work—but *dharma* specifically places career and work as well as the other roles we play in the world, within a larger context of *serving* the universe of which we are a part.

The term *dharma* is often thought to be synonymous with *profession*. People often tell me, "I don't know what my *dharma* is," when really what they mean is that they haven't yet found the career or line of work that they believe will make them happiest. *Dharma* does include what you do for a living, but it addresses more than that: it is about discovering your soul's innate and unique mission or purpose.

This larger sense of *dharma* is at the heart of the soul's inherent longing to fulfill its individual potential. Arthur Avalon, one of the world's greatest authorities on tantra, described the drive to fulfill our *dharma* as "that course of meritorious action by which man fits himself for this world, heaven, and liberation." In other words, the inherent drive or desire for *dharma* is to fully realize everything that we are capable of and, in so doing, positively affect the world. According to the tradition, there is nothing in Nature that is not compelled by this same imperative.

The reason *dharma* is the first of the four desires is twofold. One, the Vedic tradition is founded on the principle that, as individuals, our happiness is completely dependent on us fulfilling our own unique version of duty. The second reason is that everyone's unique *dharma* determines the scope and specifics of our three other desires.

> . . . .
> *The inherent drive or desire for* dharma *is to fully realize everything that we are capable of. . . . There is nothing in Nature that is not compelled by this same imperative.*
> . . . .

Artha

The second desire, *artha,* is for the means necessary to accomplish your *dharma.* In the most basic sense, *artha* refers to material resources, such as money, food, physical well-being, and a roof over your head, without which fulfilling your purpose would be difficult if not impossible. The particulars and the scope of what each of us will need to fulfill our drive for *artha* will vary from individual to individual, but all of us, even monks, have some material needs. However, *artha* is not confined to material wealth or abundance. The desire for *artha* includes all the means necessary to fulfill your soul's destiny. Mahatma Gandhi's *artha* included fasting, meditation and prayer, passive resistance, vegetarianism, even the clothes he wore, for which he spun the yarn himself. All these elements were unique to his version of *artha.* Compare him to Jackie Robinson, for example, the first African American baseball player to break the color barrier and play in the major leagues. Aside from a salary, food, and a place to sleep, some of his means included boundless will and an extraordinary capacity to endure prejudice (like Gandhi) as well as being a great baseball player. Yes, Jackie Robinson's skills on the field were a crucial part of his *artha,* the means by which he fulfilled his *dharma.*

Kama

The third desire, *kama,* is for pleasure. *Kama* is often interpreted to mean "sensuality" or "lust," but the deeper understanding of it that comes from the ancient tradition speaks of *kama* as the desire for pleasure of all kinds, including closeness and intimacy, beauty, family, art, and friendship, as well as sex. For some people there is a temptation to write this desire off as lowly or sinful, but consider whether any of us would exist if there were no desire for the pleasure of sex. If sex was not pleasurable, there is a good chance none of us would be here.

The truth is that the desire for pleasure is the motivation behind all actions. Anything and everything aspired to and achieved produces a feeling of pleasure. The following two quotes that Alain Daniélou cites from the *Mahabharata*, one of India's most revered ancient texts, make this crystal clear: "He who does not desire pleasure will not seek to enrich himself. Without desires, neither does a man desire to fulfill his duty," and "The merchant, the laborer, the gods themselves act only if their actions are linked to some satisfaction. For pleasure, a courageous man will brave the ocean." Thus, if it were not for *kama*, few things of value in this world would exist.

Moksha

The fourth and final desire, *moksha,* is the longing for liberation, true freedom. It is the intrinsic desire to realize a state free from all boundaries, including the limitations of the other three desires. This desire has been the driving force behind the world's spiritual traditions. It is the longing to know the Eternal, that which is beyond all limitations, beyond the province of the five senses and even death. It is the impulse that compels us to seek out prayer, meditation, contemplation, surrender. The desire for *moksha* is the longing for lasting peace or to experience the sacred, whether it is found in church, temple, mosque, contemplative solitude, Nature, or self-inquiry. In practical terms, *moksha* is the longing to be free, to experience unfettered awareness, to be completely unburdened. It is the aspiration to be free of suffering and realize something beyond temporal pleasure. Fulfilling this desire gives you entry into the rarest and most sublime heights—heaven on earth.

It is critical to understand that learning to honor all four desires is key to achieving both kinds of fulfillment. While *dharma* is preeminent in that it shapes the particulars of your other three desires, no one of the four is greater or more important than the rest.

At various stages of life, a particular desire often comes to the forefront as the one that needs to be focused on and fulfilled. During a health crisis, for example, *artha*—your soul's innate desire for well-being and health—would very likely become your preeminent desire. Once you regained your health, you could expect your soul to move on and place greater emphasis on fulfilling one of the other three desires. Collectively, the four desires are the compelling force that your soul utilizes to lead you to realize your full potential to become who you are meant to be.

The next part of the book, Part II, marks the beginning of the actual process of *The Four Desires*. In it I will walk you through the systematic process I've designed to find your soul's abiding purpose, recognizing your soul's purpose, and then committing to making it your guiding principle. This will chart the course to a life of lasting fulfillment that you and only you are here to achieve.

REFLECTIONS ON WARRIOR II POSE

· · · ·

Virabhadrasana II

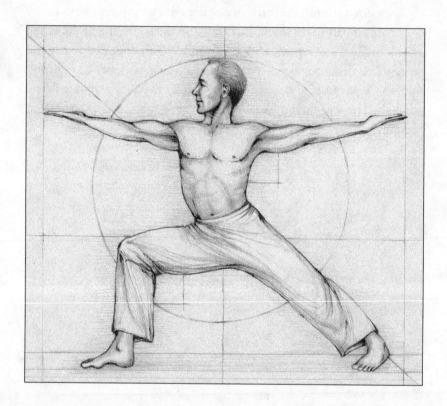

The *asana* with which I've chosen to end this first part is a powerful and enlivening standing pose that can help you navigate the fine line that separates thriving from merely being alive. Despite its appearance as a "big" and energetic pose, Warrior II is as much about internal power as physical strength. It is both grounding and expansive; it strengthens as much as it awakens a sense of grace and openness.

The foundation of Warrior II pose, like all standing postures, is the legs and feet. With the front knee bent, we sink our hips, thus fully engaging both legs, building strength in the quadriceps of the front (or bent) leg and toning the muscles of the back (straight) leg and buttocks. With this as the foundation of the pose, our focus turns toward expanding: opening the chest, spreading the arms, lifting the waist and abdomen, and lengthening the spine. The pose ultimately becomes an invitation to fully and completely expand both the body and the mind and thereby enliven the essential qualities that inspire us to grow, thrive, and evolve. It is important to see, however, that the source of growth and passion that the pose evokes is not found in a particular body part or even in the body as a whole; it is in the mind.

Essentially, to deepen into the fullest expression of the pose we must call upon internal drive and commitment. Through consistent focus and work with the breath we find greater mastery of the pose unfolding in the tiniest of increments: our spine grows taller, our breastbone lifts higher, our shoulders soften, and our eyes gaze more effortlessly. With each subtle shift and adjustment, we find ourselves becoming more present. And we find that no matter how many times we practice this posture, or any posture, the process of growth is never-ending. No matter how long you practice—years or even decades—you sense that there will always be something to learn, something more to embrace about yourself and life.

While the physical foundation for Warrior II is the earth and the legs, the psychological foundation for it is the commitment to excel—a resolve to be nothing less than fully your best self. Warrior II invites you to embody the boundless expanse of spirit and thereby prepares you to gracefully face whatever challenges stand in the way of prospering completely.

PART II

LIVE YOUR
MIGHTY PURPOSE

CHAPTER 4

. . . .

DHARMA

A Tree Bends Toward the Light

A seed settles into the soil and waits. Once it germinates, it moves stone and earth to tunnel the shoot that will become its roots. The seed projects a second shoot skyward, which will allow it to convert sunlight into the energy it will use to sustain itself for the rest of its life. Drawing upon every resource available, a seed is compelled to become the thing it was meant to be: tree, grass, vine, bush, shrub, or flower. If unsuccessful, it will have died trying, but not before exhausting every last fiber of its being to fulfill its potential.

A honeybee, drawing nectar from a blossom, bats its wings at 11,400 times per minute. Salmon swim as much as a thousand miles upstream, or more, in order to spawn. An ant will carry twenty times its weight to serve a colony. This same drive, all but invisible, pervades everything in the natural world. The world we live in is little more than an endless and vibrant expression of energy.

In material terms, this energy fuels the extraordinary feats that make life possible. Linda Acredolo and Susan Goodwyn write that human "fetal cells destined to become brain cells begin to multiply at the astonishing rate of about 250,000 per minute. . . . By the time a baby makes her debut into the world, she will have an astronomical number of brain cells . . . a mind-boggling 100 to 200 billion." The ocean's total energy flux, at any given moment, has been estimated to be a force equal to 280 trillion watt-hours. A solar flare—a release of magnetic energy in the solar atmosphere—is equivalent to millions of 100-megaton hydrogen bombs exploding at the same time.

From the microscopic to the cosmic, our world is a vibrant place, but it is shaped by more than sheer force. It is under the constant care and guidance of a kind of intelligence or order. Thus a tree bends toward light—always. Responding to the shortening of days, a tree drops its leaves and becomes dormant; once spring arrives and the days grow longer again, it produces new buds. Humpback whales migrate thousands of miles to breed and calve, and they stay there until, just as their food supply has been replenished, something prompts them to return to their original home.

Similarly, human life transitions from zygote to embryo, newborn, infant, child, adolescent, and adult—always. An embryologist can predict and describe in great detail each stage of development of a human embryo because, under normal circumstances, like every other developing organism, it develops according to a highly organized and predictable pattern.

The first time I saw a film using time-lapse photography, I was in second or third grade. In the short film, several weeks were compressed into a little less than a minute. I watched, transfixed, as a small cut on someone's thumb healed, transitioning from bloody laceration through stages of scabbing into what would finally be completely restored flesh with hardly any trace of a scar. This sped-up version made it seem like the healing process was a seamless and effortless undertaking. Eventually I would learn that it was anything but: in order to heal even the tiniest cut millions of separate microscopic events have to take place, all of which must work in perfect coordination with each other before their collective goal of healing will be achieved.

What is it that allows the infinite number of events that take place within Nature to work in such an orderly way? What is it that, in combination with the inherent force of Nature, informs all of these life processes to work in concert?

The Vedic tradition addresses these questions. Indeed, the study of what compels and organizes the myriad events of Nature, and how human beings fit into its scheme, is at the very heart of the Vedic exploration of the universe.

According to the tradition, an abiding intelligence works with the forces of Nature to orchestrate all of Nature's countless actions, including the healing of your body. This intelligence or force pervades and informs everything, from the functioning of a single cell to the pulsation of the most distant star. It is the invisible fabric that binds everything together into one seamless whole.

Max Planck, the father of quantum mechanics, described it this way: "All matter originates and exists only by virtue of a force. . . . We must assume behind this force the existence of a conscious and intelligent mind. This mind is the matrix of all matter."

The Vedic tradition has a word for this invisible intelligence that sustains and organizes all forms of life. It is *dharma*. In Part I we saw that the word *dharma* was used to identify the first and most preeminent of the four desires—the longing for purpose and to fulfill our unique destiny. However, the Vedic tradition also uses the term to identify an even more far-reaching concept.

> . . . .
> *We are each a single cell in the greater body of this world, with a unique role to play in the service of sustaining and advancing the whole of which we are a part.*
> . . . .

The root of the word *dharma* is *dri,* which means "to support" or "to hold up." In its largest context, *dharma* is the unseen and limitless web of intelligence that sustains and supports both the universe as a whole and each individual creation (person, plant, animal, even mineral) within it. Every cell in your body is sustained by *dharma,* and at the same time, *dharma* organizes and guides all the various kinds of cells (liver, heart, lungs, kidney, bone, and so on) in your body to carry out their unique roles and, in so doing, to act collectively to support the functioning of your whole body. In a similar fashion, *dharma* supports you, as an individual, in your role as an essential part of the whole of life. In this sense we are each a single cell in the greater body of this world, with a unique role to play in the service of sustaining and advancing the whole of which we are a part.

Thus, besides referring to the intelligence that pervades the universe, *dharma* is the compelling force in each of us that longs to thrive, to become who and what we are meant to be. Furthermore, the principle of *dharma* asserts that what is in our true best interest as an individual (microcosm) is necessarily in the best interest of the universe (macrocosm). As Arthur Avalon writes, *dharma* is "the eternal and immutable principles," that "hold together the universe in its parts and in its whole." It is, in the end, the "principle of right living."

The theme of living in harmony with our *dharma* and the subtle world of which we are all a part is the foundation of Vedic and yogic philosophy. Although the spiritual teachings of India are commonly referred to as Hinduism, they were and still are rightfully referred to as *sanantana dharma*. *Sanantana* means "infinite," "eternal"; thus *sanantana dharma* means "eternal law" or "the way of the Eternal." *Sanantana dharma* conveys the abiding spirit of the ancient teachings—the idea that there is a collective natural order of which we are all a part. We all come from and are sustained by this all-pervading and limitless intelligence.

Albert Einstein observed that a human being is part of a whole, called by us "universe," a part limited in time and space. He experiences his thoughts and feelings as something separate from the rest—a kind of optical delusion of his consciousness. This delusion is a kind of prison for us, restricting us to our personal desires and to affection for a few people near us. Our task must be to free ourselves from this prison by widening our circle of compassion to embrace all living creatures and the whole of Nature in its beauty.

Einstein's incisive words convey the core principle of *dharma*. The ancient tradition does indeed ask us to widen our vision and to see beyond the perception that we are separate from everything else. If ever there was a definitive philosophy for lasting happiness, Einstein managed to capture it. The principle of *dharma* is the enduring truth that individual happiness is inextricably linked to the fate of the world around us. We see this, for example, in the way all of us affect the air that we breathe and the water we drink, even the food we eat, and the way that all of the economies in the world are interrelated. Given our increased awareness of events around the world as they happen and of our ever-increasing global interdependence, there may never have been a more crucial time to ask ourselves how we can achieve our individual happiness while simultaneously having a positive impact on the world of which we are a part.

This is not to suggest that we give up wanting things for ourselves or avoid seeking to better ourselves; in fact, as we've seen, the opposite is true. The Vedic tradition makes it clear that when we act based on our highest aspirations, we contribute to and elevate the best interests of the sum total of all. The point is that if you are committed to achieving true and lasting happiness, it is vital to learn how to recognize the intrinsic desires of your soul, which are forever linked to the guidance and intelligence of *dharma*.

This teaching is, in fact, the centerpiece of the yoga tradition. Nowhere is this more clearly brought to light than in India's most widely revered spiritual scripture, the Bhagavad Gita. While spanning the entirety of human experience, the essential theme of the Gita can be boiled down to this: act and shape yourself and life according to the innate wisdom that sustains this world. If you do, you will be happy; if you don't, you won't. In other words, fulfillment is realized by aligning the ways you act, think, and speak with the infinite intelligence that pervades all things. Suffering, on the other hand, is the result of not being in harmony with this universal intelligence. In the context of the Gita, yoga is the means by which we become able to fully align ourselves with, and respond to, *dharma*.

The Gita tells us we live in a world where we confront many challenges and face many choices. Learning to see the path that will lead us to the greatest happiness is not always easy. Therefore, the ancient sages counseled that we practice yoga to still our minds so that we can discern how best to fulfill our personal *dharma*—the one and only key to lasting happiness.

Throughout the ages, human beings have felt drawn to understand their place in the larger scheme of life or *dharma*. We seem to have always intuitively known that the more we can understand and embody this force or intelligence, the more capable we will become and the more our lives will reflect the fullness of *dharma*'s endless power and capacity. Thus we seek it out in countless ways.

Marveling at a newborn child's smile or a toddler's first steps is a window into the profound and hidden mystery of *dharma*. We know instinctively that we are watching something extraordinary, something timeless, unfold. Indeed, millions of unseen events are taking place, which together are responsible for that child taking shape in an utterly unique way and yet in a way that is uncannily the same as all the other children who have come before and will come after. Behind it all we sense that there is an intelligence, a drive to be and to become. We are sensing *dharma*, expressing itself in this unique and adorable human being's desire to become who and what it is meant to be.

Whether or not we are aware of it, watching a young child provides an opportunity to glimpse our connection to an intelligence greater than ourselves. Mystics of all cultures and religious traditions have understood this. That is why they are so deeply committed to being able to "see" or commune with that which connects all of life. However, the desire to commune with infinite intelligence is not the sole domain of mystics. A skilled surfer seeks it out as he or she paddles into the ocean's surging power just as it is peaking into a wave. The "perfect ride" provides a tactile thrill, but at another level the exaltation comes from being connected to, at one with, what Max Planck described as the "matrix of all matter"—which at that moment happens to be expressing itself as a wave in the ocean. A similar experience awaits the skilled gardener who plies soil, seed, sun, and water into beauty, color, or sustenance. Artists, engineers, mathematicians, musicians, and yogis also seek communion with this intelligence. Each, in his or her own way, is drawn to understand, express, or directly commune with this sublime intelligence that shapes our world. Being touched or in some way moved by *dharma* is something we have all felt.

You may have sensed it in the awe-inspiring cascade of a waterfall, or in the quiet, still, vibrant presence of a century-old oak tree, or the vast expanse of the ocean. It is the power that fills the ineffable beauty of silence.

This intelligence and power abounds in Nature, but if you have ever stood in St. Peter's Basilica in Rome or beside the Great Pyramids in Egypt, you may have felt it as well. It is as alive beneath the hubbub of New York City as it is in the Serengeti plains of Africa. There is, however, an important distinction between how this most basic power manifests in Nature and how it manifests in human beings. It is practically impossible to find anything in Nature that fails to completely embody the power of *dharma* to its fullest. Even the tiniest plant, for example, in the most challenging of circumstances, will exhaust every ounce of its energy to thrive. On the other hand, human beings sometimes choose to do otherwise. We can and often do stray from our innate impulse to fulfill all of our potential.

Perhaps this is why we are so moved by those who choose to live exceptional lives and by those who overcome disability, tragedy, or challenging circumstances. Beethoven's Ninth Symphony, for example, is moving because of the grandeur of its vision and expression as a piece of music, but listening to it while knowing that it was composed by someone who was unable to hear the masterpiece he had created makes it that much more moving to me. I can't help being touched by the greatness of the human spirit that it expresses and that gave birth to it. The world's great athletes are revered not just for their natural talents but for the force of will that enables them to accomplish great things. In cheering for them, we are at some level cheering for the part of ourselves that aspires to become everything we are capable of becoming.

> . . . .
> *Your long-term happiness and fulfillment depend on your ability to fulfill your personal* dharma *and fill the place in the world that only you can fill.*
> . . . .

In our more lucid moments, when we have quieted the hubbub of our distractions, we are capable of sensing the power and intelligence that sustain us and everything else. In such moments, it is hard not to feel touched by the sublime, by that which links all the things in the world together, by the eternal essence that is at the heart of our existence.

The principle of eternal law is the foundation of Vedic wisdom and *The Four Desires.* The essential points of eternal law are concisely outlined by my teacher Pandit Rajmani Tigunait in his book *Freedom from Fear:*

- Life is inherently sacred.
- There is a clear and definite order to the world you live in.
- By honoring your place in it—your individual *dharma*—you honor and, in the process, support, universal *dharma.*
- Since you affect the larger *dharma* through your actions, thoughts, and words, nothing is more important than securing and establishing your highest state of well-being so that you can be more completely in tune with this intelligence.

In other words, you can thrive only when you live in ways that are in harmony with the intelligence of which you are a part. Your long-term happiness and fulfillment depend on your ability to fulfill your personal *dharma* and fill the place in the world that only you can fill, making the contribution that only you can make. Aligning yourself with the intelligence of the universe means coming to understand your life's purpose and living your life in such a way that you are manifesting this purpose through all four desires.

CHAPTER 5

· · · ·

UNDERSTANDING *YOUR* MIGHTY PURPOSE

A profound dedication to purpose defined the lives of Socrates, Lao Tzu, St. Francis of Assisi, Michelangelo, Susan B. Anthony, Florence Nightingale, Frederick Douglass, Marie Curie, Frank Lloyd Wright, Winston Churchill, Eleanor Roosevelt, and Nelson Mandela. All of them, in their unique way, embodied the power of *dharma* by connecting to their life purpose. St. Francis of Assisi's dedication to his life purpose to be a beacon of Christ's light in the world inspired his founding of the Franciscan order of monks. Florence Nightingale's dedication to her life purpose to heal inspired her to revolutionize the concept and practice of nursing. Nelson Mandela's dedication to his life purpose led to the end of apartheid in South Africa.

By connecting to your life purpose, you gather the forces of Nature in the same way a seed does when it starts to germinate. Great, sometimes even miraculous-seeming achievements become possible when you are doing something with your life that you know in your innermost heart is truly meaningful. Anyone you can think of who has achieved something of real, lasting, and positive significance has had this kind of connection to a profound sense of purpose.

The Dharma Code

My intention is to help you access this same force of *dharma,* and once you do, to help you manifest it through any or all four of your desires. To do this, I will help you uncover what I call your Dharma Code, your unique life purpose, and then help you put it into words. Your Dharma Code conveys in very clear and direct language the life course that your soul aspires to, the one you were meant to follow. The rationale for finding your Dharma Code is a simple one: the moment you discover and commit to serving your Dharma Code, you begin the process of being lifted into the power of your soul and connecting with unbridled strength, courage, and enthusiasm. You become a force of Nature. When you know and choose to serve your Dharma Code—your soul's driving reason for being—you are able to collect and channel extraordinary power into your life because you are then linked to the infinite field of energy and intelligence that shapes the world. Once you are rooted in your soul's defining purpose, you will be able to use your Dharma Code to direct every action and decision from the light of your soul. Your Dharma Code will also enable you to determine which of your desires are essential and can lead you to your highest destiny, and which will not.

I want to make it clear that by defining your life purpose, your Dharma Code, you are not trying to create a list of specific goals. Whereas goals come and go, a Dharma Code endures, remaining constant through all of your life's circumstances. Your Dharma Code will be your guiding principle for all four desires, not just the first desire, *dharma,* which focuses on your career path or the way you directly contribute to the world at large. Your Dharma Code also informs you about the second desire, *artha* (the means, including money, health, and material security), the third, *kama* (pleasure in all areas of life), and finally the fourth, *moksha* (true freedom and spiritual awakening). By connecting you to the one thing that all four of your desires are meant to serve, your Dharma Code is your key to the door of lasting happiness.

"The key to happiness is very simple," Swami Rama would often say. "First, become clear what your duty or purpose is in life. Second, learn to love it." These few words encapsulate one of the essential principles of the Vedic tradition—the idea that each and every one of us is born with a glorious purpose. According to the ancient teachings, your soul's unique purpose—your Dharma Code—is hardwired. It is not something you consciously decide. Your soul's purpose came into this world with you, even if you are not yet aware of it. It has always been a part of you. It's up to you to uncover it—to bring it to a conscious level—and then make living by it your priority.

Swami Rama's advice summarizes the guidance that Lord Krishna offers his devotee Arjuna in the Bhagavad Gita. "It is better to perform one's own duties [*dharma*] imperfectly than to master the duties of another. By fulfilling the obligations he is born with, a person never comes to grief. No one should abandon duties [*dharma*] because he sees defects in them." Why? Because, as I've said, you can never be completely at peace if you are not fulfilling your own purpose. However, before you can fulfill your purpose, you need to know what it is.

> . . . .
> *Great, sometimes even miraculous-seeming achievements become possible when you are doing something with your life that you know in your innermost heart is truly meaningful.*
> . . . .

George Bernard Shaw, the Nobel Prize winner and renowned social, political, and theatrical critic who died at the age of ninety-four and whose plays are some of the most widely acclaimed and produced in the English language, echoed this underlying teaching of the Gita when he wrote, "This is the true joy in life, the being used for a purpose recognized by yourself as a mighty one . . . ; the being a force of Nature instead of a feverish selfish little clod of ailments and grievances complaining that the world will not devote itself to making you happy." Notice that Shaw said "being used *for* a purpose." Shaw recognized that your job as a human being, the joy in life, is to serve your soul's "mighty" purpose. You will find joy and real fulfillment in life only when you find a mighty purpose to serve.

Benjamin Franklin weighed in with a similar view for living and achieving a supreme life: "The masterpiece of man, is to live to the purpose." Add Paramahansa Yogananda, the world-famous author of *Autobiography of a Yogi,* to the list of those who praised the power and significance of finding and living your purpose. "Analyze what you are," he wrote in *The Law of Success,* "what you wish to become, and what shortcomings are impeding you. Decide the nature of your true task— your mission in life. Endeavor to make yourself what you should be and what you want to be."

In their comments about the key to a fulfilled life, Swami Rama, Shaw, Benjamin Franklin, and Paramahansa Yogananda are all reflecting the heart of Vedic wisdom and the core teaching of the Bhagavad Gita: the moment you fully commit to something supremely purposeful that is resonant or in harmony with the larger scheme of your life, your life changes irrevocably for the better. Why? Because the moment you marry yourself to the right purpose you become, as Shaw described it, "a force of nature."

When you complete the process described in the following chapters, you will have uncovered your soul's unique purpose and you will have established a foundation for achieving your best life—the one that you came into this world to fulfill and that is your most rewarding and most glorious destiny.

A Foundation for Lasting Happiness: Laura's Story

Laura had studied with me for several years before she met with me for a personal consultation. The moment our session started, before I could say a word, she began weeping. Fighting through tears, she told me that her "heart had been broken." The man she was in love with had abruptly ended their relationship. She then began recounting their endless struggles as a couple. She spoke at length about their troubled relationship and how it escalated to his verbal and emotional abuse. The more I heard, the worse their relationship sounded, and the less I understood why she was heartbroken that it had ended.

She was still crying when she finally stopped talking. "Laura," I asked, "what kept you in the relationship? Did you make any effort to tell him to stop treating you that way?"

"No," she replied.

"Why would you let yourself be treated so badly and not end it yourself or at least speak up for yourself and draw boundaries of what was acceptable behavior?"

"I've always been afraid of telling the truth. I'll admit to you," she went on, "I've always felt like a scolded child."

The words "scolded child" jumped out at me.

"I've never been good at speaking up for myself," she added.

With that as our starting point, I learned that Laura, in her mid-forties, had never had a long-term relationship. She had grown up with elderly parents. Her much older sister had already left home by the time Laura was born. From what I could gather, Laura must have been an unwelcome late-life surprise, to parents who wanted her to be heard and seen as little as possible. No wonder Laura rarely spoke up for herself; she had grown up in a home where doing so was discouraged. Laura had never ventured far from either the geographic or the emotional confines of her childhood. She remained near the same small town she grew up in, and long after her parents passed away she continued to feel like the invisible, unheard child they had trained her to be.

My strategy for helping someone move through her or his life issues is rooted in the yogic idea that a part of us is always free and that life is an endless landscape with infinite possibilities. We all have some negative or destructive memories; however, yoga teaches that we do not have to be at their mercy. Thus I focus less on helping people understand the whys of self-limiting and self-destructive behaviors and more on guiding them to the ways to overcome such behaviors. In Laura's case, this meant I was less interested in dwelling on the life experiences that had led to her problematic relationships and more focused on helping her find a foothold for acting in a way that would help her thrive—to find the freedom and power she needed to create more of the life she wanted, including a loving relationship.

I asked Laura if there was ever a time when she thrived, when she felt free, unburdened by doubt or by the fear of speaking up for herself. Without any hesitation, she responded, "When I teach. When I'm teaching, I feel absolutely free." Laura taught part-time at the university level. She had been a teacher for more than two decades and was also a tireless volunteer in various community outreach services. As she spoke about teaching and volunteering, it was impossible not to notice a dramatic shift in her demeanor. More than just relieved to be talking about something that brought her joy, she was speaking and acting like a different person—truly lighthearted and purposeful. Teaching was a place where she gave herself permission to be fully herself.

"Clearly you don't feel afraid when you teach," I said. "I'm curious, Laura. Can you tell me what your intention is when you teach? I am hoping you can identify the intention that allows you to overcome your fears when you are teaching."

Laura shrugged. She had no idea what I was asking.

"You communicate freely when you're teaching," I went on, "and you seem to have a great time doing it. But intimate relationships are challenging for you. While both teaching and intimate relationships require you to interact with others, in one area, you thrive; in the other, you have difficulty. I believe you have one intention when you teach and a very different intention when you're in a serious relationship. Let's figure out what your intention is when you teach because that is where you feel free."

It was a challenge getting Laura to understand what I was asking for, but when she finally got it, it was like watching a light go on. "When I teach, my intention is to share. I just share all of myself."

Yes, she had found exactly what I was asking her to pinpoint! She had identified the intention that shaped her approach to teaching. She continued, "Without thinking about it and without worrying about the consequences, whether I am teaching senior citizens or freshmen in college, I just share."

"Laura," I asked, "what do you think would happen if you were to make 'I just share all of myself' the sole purpose of your life? In other words, what if you applied it to each and every situation of your life, including your next intimate relationship?"

> • • • •
>
> *The foundation for lasting happiness and fulfillment is finding and living your life's purpose.*
>
> • • • •

I watched Laura carefully considering what I was proposing.

"You have identified a purpose or overarching intention that, when you apply it, allows you to thrive," I told her. "The ancient teachings suggest that we are all born with a unique purpose to fulfill and that our happiness is determined by how completely we allow it to shape our lives. 'I just share all of myself' may well be your soul's purpose or Dharma Code. It would not surprise me at all if it *is*. Very often our Dharma Code is the driving force behind the things that give us the most joy *and* also is behind our recurring challenges—the ones we often need to work through as part of the life lessons we are here to learn.

"For the time being, why not assume that 'I just share all of myself' is your Dharma Code and commit to letting it guide your actions, thoughts, and speech? Do it at work, at the checkout stand at the market, when you write e-mails, when you run in marathons, when you come to yoga seminars, and in your relationships—all of them. The critical point is that you've got to let 'I just share all of myself' burn brighter than your fear. It's important to realize that in the past you've applied 'I just share all of myself,' but in only one area of your life—when you are teaching. I'm asking you to make it your whole life's mission, to make it your soul's credo, which you will always honor and act upon in every situation in your life."

As I spoke, I could see Laura imagining her life propelled by this singular idea. Sensing what it might be like to spend her life in the same place she lived in when she taught had an almost immediate, palpable effect. The person who twenty minutes earlier had been in tears describing her life now looked joyful and inspired. A part of her clearly loved the idea of letting this particular defining purpose guide her. She had a real sense that what I was suggesting could provide her with a path to a future very different from the life she had been leading.

Laura and I went on to discuss her practice. "Share all of yourself. Make sharing all of yourself—good, bad, or indifferent—the primary focus of your life," I said, "and please share the results of your efforts with me. In three months send me an e-mail and tell me if and how it's made a difference." Before our session was over, I made one more recommendation: meditation. I prescribed a specific practice to help her build self-reliance and self-trust (you'll find this practice, the Healing the Heart Meditation, described in detail in Part IV).

A few months later I received the following e-mail from Laura.

Dear Rod,

The practice of keeping my Dharma Code always in mind—to just share all of myself—has truly turned my life around. It has helped me make sense of loose threads that I always knew were there. It's moved me to finally make richer and more meaningful contact and dialogue with others (friends, students, strangers, and who knows what to come . . .), the very stuff that for most of my life seemed impossibly beyond reach.

Many years of off-and-on therapy with some fantastic therapists helped my soul out of its hole many times, but somehow being conscious of and living with the guidance of my Dharma Code has done that sort of work in a way that not only "sticks better," but that feels utterly genuine, truthful, and empowering. That is probably because it's not just about finding a way to make myself feel less pain; it is about sharing myself with others and using those "aha" moments to better illuminate both them and my self.

I am aware of a difference in the way others are looking at me. The practice is ingraining me so that when my next lover appears, I will not settle for anything less than being fully myself.

Thank you, so much.

Warm regards,

Laura

It's been four years since our meeting. I'm pleased to be able to say that Laura has been in a relationship for more than a year. She is with a man who is kind and nurturing, and they are very much in love. However, having intimacy and love in her life is only one facet of Laura's metamorphosis, and it did not happen immediately. What did happen soon after our meeting is that her life as a whole became fuller and richer than it had ever been. Uncovering and living her purpose—to share all of herself—became a foundation that inspired and transformed the way she thought and acted. It enabled her to live her life in an entirely different way. She was freer, lighter, more self-confident. Her commitment to serving her higher purpose empowered her to express more of who she was and what she aspired to be, to take risks, and to show up for herself in ways that she had never even imagined. Laura moved across the country, began teaching full-time, and expanded her social circle. Eventually her commitment to letting her purpose guide and shape her life led her to the loving relationship that she had spent most of her life doubting she would ever have.

Laura's story provides *the* essential lesson for anyone wanting a truly fulfilled life: the foundation for lasting happiness and fulfillment is finding and living your life's purpose.

You Choose Your Destiny

My first teacher, Mani, was the one who first opened my eyes to the power of *dharma.*

Mani was a commanding presence. His impassioned way of speaking and his booming voice made it nearly impossible not to take notice of everything he said. "You are responsible for your life," he roared, lecturing a group of us one night. "The sooner you see how you have determined your fate, the sooner and more completely you will have the life you want." I understood his point, but the more I thought about it, the more I found myself questioning it. My mind wandered to many of the difficulties that I had had to contend with through no fault of my own: my parents' separation and subsequent divorce when I was a child; being raised by a single mother who had less money than most of the parents whose children I grew up with; having a father who was someone I was in awe of from afar more than a real or loving presence in my life. The more I considered it, the more convinced I became that I had had little to do with the circumstances determining my fate, and the more Mani's statement bothered me. It certainly wasn't a particularly enlightened or compassionate view of the world, I thought, reflecting on the lives of other people I knew whose circumstances were far less fortunate than mine, also through no fault of their own.

My attention drifted back to Mani's words just in time to hear him acknowledge that no one controls all the circumstances in which they find themselves. Hurricanes, earthquakes, fires, misfortune, blighted childhoods, abuse, war, and disease are not things that anyone consciously chooses. "However," he continued, holding to his point, "because you choose how you will respond to these circumstances, it is *you* and *only you* who, in the end, has and will determine your destiny."

I left the lecture that night with the words "You are responsible for your life" bouncing in my head. It would be a while before I would come to accept them completely. Decades later I see the principles that he was teaching as one of the most valuable lessons that Mani, or anyone, has ever given me.

At the heart of it is a truth so universal and so simple that I believe you can never achieve the life of your dreams—a life of real meaning and purpose—until you fully grasp it and live it: the core of a fulfilled life is knowing that every moment is a *choice*.

Eventually, upon deeper reflection, I saw that Mani was right: I, more than my circumstances, determine who and what I am and will be. I am the sum of everything I choose to do, think, and say: how many cups of tea I drink a day; the way I talk to my wife and my kids; what I read; how I relieve stress; the people with whom I spend my time; if I watch television and what I watch; the number of hours I work; what I do every morning upon waking; whether or not I floss. Life is little more than an endless series of moments strung together by a single thread—choice.

> *The destiny you have achieved up until now has been shaped by all the choices you have made in the past.*

As decisions big and small accumulate minute by minute, year by year, they gradually shape a particular fate. You may not recognize that you are always making choices, but that doesn't change the fact that you are, and the destiny you have achieved up until now has been shaped by all the choices you have made in the past.

Admittedly, the world and the people in it are not always just; yet the more you blame factors outside yourself—your parents, genetics, "enemies," taxes, God, conservatives or liberals, the people who betrayed or took advantage of you, your boss, bad drivers, the subway system, the overcommercialization of Christmas, or anything else—the more you dilute your power and weaken your ability to shape the life toward which your soul is intent on guiding you.

Your choices, much more than your circumstances, determine who and what you are.

It is vital to see that the process by which you will shape your ideal future is the sum of the choices you make. From a seemingly infinite array of desires, you will choose to pursue some desires and ignore others. What determines which desires you'll choose to act on and which ones you will not choose to act on? The answer is your deepest driving desire.

"You are what your deep, driving desire is," says the *Brihadaranyaka Upanishad.* "As your desire is, so is your will. As your will is, so is your deed. As your deed is, so is your destiny." In other words, by determining your will and your actions, your deepest driving desire is, above all else, what actually determines your fate.

When your deepest driving desire is in harmony with your soul's purpose, it guides you toward fulfilling the promise of who you are meant to be. However, when your deepest driving desire is something other than, or in conflict with, your soul's purpose, it may cause you to make choices that work against that purpose without being aware of it.

Laura is a case in point. It's important to see that before we had uncovered her Dharma Code, she, like all of us, had a deepest driving desire. However, it was *not* the one that would carry her to the life her soul truly aspired to. Until our meeting, Laura's deepest driving desire had been something like "to not be heard or seen." This deepest driving desire was not coming from her soul; it was coming from the beliefs imposed on her in childhood. But it had nonetheless determined her fate. If she was ever going to have a different fate, she would have to find and then learn to serve a different deepest driving desire.

Without ever using the term Dharma Code at the time, I had walked Laura through an expedited version of the process for uncovering one. Shortly after we discovered hers and she began acting on it, Laura changed her destiny.

It should be clear to you by now that your life is shaped by your most deeply held intentions. If you are going to manifest your most auspicious life—the one that's going to bring you the most happiness and satisfaction—it is vital to clarify your soul's priorities and commit to them.

CHAPTER 6

. . . .

WHAT IS *YOUR* DHARMA CODE?

As we've seen, the Dharma Code is each person's individual expression of his or her *dharma* or soul's purpose. It is a statement that clarifies your soul's reason for being. When acted upon, it is a principle that will benefit not just your own *dharma,* but the larger or universal expression of it as well. In uncovering and articulating your Dharma Code, you will be providing the opportunity for your soul to direct you to be more fully yourself and, in so doing, contribute more effectively to the benefit of the world.

Anne Frank once wrote, "I want to be useful or bring enjoyment to all people, even those I've never met. I want to go on living even after my death!" As most of us know, Anne Frank would later die in a Nazi concentration camp. Yet she did in fact fulfill her intention. Long past her death, her words, wisdom, and life experience continue to uplift those she never met, enabling her to achieve her dream of usefulness to others and immortality. It is well documented that Anne Frank wanted to be a writer, but underlying that specific desire was a deeper and more profound aim, which her writing helped her to achieve. This remarkable and brave young woman seemed to know her life's purpose—her Dharma Code.

Human beings are able to overcome the most extraordinary challenges, particularly when they feel connected to, guided, or supported by something larger than themselves. Armed with the resolve to "live to the purpose," as Benjamin Franklin put it, you become more courageous, more patient, more capable, and more imaginative. You are able to generate indomitable willpower and determination.

Your Dharma Code, in addition to helping to propel you toward living your fullest life possible, has two other very practical uses and a third that might be considered more mystical. First, it will serve as an anchor, helping you remain true to your vision of your best self whenever conflict or confusion arises. Second, as you will see in Part III, it will act as a general guide to all future life decisions, helping you identify and prioritize specific, personal short-term desires. Finally, intuition and synchronicity are two more seeds that will blossom and bear fruit for you.

Anne Frank was able to sum up the aim of her life as "I want to be useful or bring enjoyment to all people, even those I've never met. I want to go on living even after my death!" A Dharma Code can be shorter or longer. "Never hesitate to know God and to be great" was the Dharma Code of one of my students. The ten-year-old daughter of another of my students, upon hearing about the Dharma Code at the dinner table one night, went around the table spontaneously declaiming what she saw as each family member's Dharma Code. When she finally got to herself, she declared that hers was, "I am the moon and you can't resist me." This confident young girl did a perfect job; she had identified and declared her soul's purpose. The point is that your Dharma Code must be an authentic expression of your soul's reason for being and has to speak directly to you, from you.

Life Change: Rob's Story

Rob was a struggling actor. Despite his good looks, considerable talent, and years of hard work, his acting jobs never amounted to the career he wanted. A friend suggested that he come to my Yoga of Fulfillment class. He was ambivalent about exploring a yogic approach to what he saw as the very practical problem of his career, but he was so frustrated creatively and financially that he came, hoping for a solution.

One of the first and most important things I ask people to consider when they are trying to uncover their Dharma Code is the question of what they want their lives to have stood for.

"What values, principles, or deep sense of purpose do you want your life to have exemplified?" I always ask. "Instead of trying to decide whether you should be an architect or an actor, a politician or a policeman, the more important thing to ask is what you want your life to embody. In other words, what truly gives your life meaning? What, deep in your heart, do you want to have contributed to the world? By the time your life is over you may or may not have achieved all your specific desires, but you always have a choice about the values you want to live by."

When Rob began to search out his deeper motivations for wanting to be an actor, he realized that acting was only a vehicle, the one that he had chosen to realize his deeper goal of inspiring people and moving them toward positive change. Deep down, Rob loved the experience of touching people's hearts, to get them to think more deeply about themselves and about their connection to the rest of humanity. This is what he ultimately hoped to achieve through acting. Doing the exercise, he put his Dharma Code into these words: "I uplift others. I provide them with experiences that inspire them to think and grow."

Rob's own willingness to think and grow, along with his maturity, allowed him to accept that fulfilling his deep-seated values was just as important to him as succeeding as an actor, perhaps even more so. That was the pivotal decision that was key to all the positive changes that were to come.

At the end of the seminar, Rob still had the goal of becoming a successful actor. However, the process of uncovering his deepest driving desire would eventually lead him in another direction. Before they left, I asked every participant to commit to a specific action, consistent with their newly discovered life purpose, that would help them establish positive momentum toward living that purpose. For a long time Rob had painted as a hobby. Over the years, he had never thought about trying to sell his work. At the time of the seminar, he had accumulated a collection of his paintings. The commitment he made was to put together a circle of other artists he knew and stage a benefit, the proceeds of which would go to a worthwhile cause. The event turned out to be a success, both in terms of the money it raised and, more important for Rob, in helping him see that his paintings could be a vehicle to fulfill his deepest goals. That was the turning point that spurred Rob to throw himself completely into painting.

In the years since, instead of pursuing an acting career Rob has become an accomplished and acclaimed artist. He never stops working. His art is truly inspiring. He finds the solitude of painting, the act of painting itself, and showing his work to be wholly fulfilling.

I should point out that Rob's transition from aspiring actor to working painter did not occur without some struggle. His commitment to becoming a full-time painter occurred only after he recognized the fact that acting afforded him so few opportunities to fulfill his soul's purpose. During this process, Rob's Dharma Code was already beginning to guide him. Nonetheless, even as it was becoming increasingly clear to him that painting was the primary vehicle for him to express his Dharma Code, he experienced sadness over the loss of the dream about acting that he had held on to for so long.

Rob gradually realized that working with his Dharma Code endowed him with a sense of clarity and direction, even during those times when he had no expectation that it could. He found that the more he consciously used his Dharma Code as a guide to making choices, the more it benefited him. As time went on, devoting himself to his new mission felt liberating; increasingly, painting gave him the sense that he was doing exactly what he was meant to be doing. Eventually, to his surprise, he didn't miss acting at all. "It was profoundly freeing to live for a purpose," he told me. "Instead of hoping for an acting job, I was being guided to take control of my life. I'd always heard about the value of nonattachment, suddenly I found myself thriving because I was living it."

Rob's story is also another illustration of how our actions more positively impact the world around us once we uncover and commit to our Dharma Code. His breakthrough touched and benefited not just him but a much larger community—everyone who comes in contact with his art and with the more fulfilled person that Rob has become. This is the exquisite and magical part of uncovering and committing to your Dharma Code. As I've said, when you learn to listen to your soul's calling and let it guide you, you honor and support the invisible web of connection that links you to the universe as a whole.

Rob's life changed because he followed the sage advice of Swami Rama—he found his life's purpose, and then he learned to love it. Doing so allowed him access to something mighty, a current whose force carried him and helped him to be and to become all that he was capable of.

Rob's transformation brings to my mind the words by the great sage and yoga master Swami Satyananda Saraswati, disciple of Sri Swami Sivananda Saraswati.

There will never be a storm
That can wash the path from my feet,
The direction from my heart,
The light from my eyes,
Or the purpose from this life.
I know that I am untouchable to the forces
As long as I have a direction, an aim, a goal:
To serve, to love, and to give.
Strength lies in the magnification of the secret qualities
Of my own personality, my own character
And though I am only a messenger,
I am me.

"To serve, to love, and to give" is what Swami Satyananda Saraswati found to be his soul's purpose. The words he found to describe it provided him a clear direction, a force that propelled him to be a beacon of contentment and inspiration to the many whose lives he touched.

He knew his soul's purpose; now it is time to for you to know yours.

THE DHARMA CODE EXERCISE

Since your Dharma Code is a statement that declares your soul's innate purpose, you are not so much *deciding* on it as you are *uncovering* it. Instead of asking you to specify your Dharma Code with your conscious mind, I strongly recommend you use the exercise below, which is designed to bypass your conscious mind and help you access a more intuitive and penetrating level of insight.

Having explored the concept and power of *dharma*, we are ready to walk through the steps for uncovering your own Dharma Code. This three-part exercise provides you with the rare opportunity to pose life's most meaningful questions directly to your soul. Your answers will soon become your foundation for a lifetime of lasting happiness.

Before you begin, a plea: Please be patient. Give yourself enough time to read the directions thoroughly before starting. It's worth it! As you read through the directions, all you will need is your imagination. When it comes time to do the exercise you will need something to write with and seven to ten sheets of paper. After you've read the overview, when you're ready to begin the actual exercise, go to a quiet place where you will not be disturbed or distracted for about an hour or so; you may not need that much time, but it's a good idea to set that much time aside just in case.

Step 1: Imagining a Life Well Lived: Your Own

The first step of this exercise is to imagine yourself celebrating a significant birthday sometime near the end of your life, at a time when you can enjoy the satisfaction of having achieved the life of your dreams. You can think of this event as occurring at any age you like. The oldest woman on record right now, Sakhan Dosova of Kazakhstan, is 130. You might not want to live that long, but then again, you might!

This ideal scenario that I'm asking you to imagine will allow you to consider what your life would look like if, from this moment forward, you lived "mightily"—investing all of yourself purposefully, materially, sensually, and spiritually toward the fulfillment of your desires.

The next step is to imagine that your closest friends, family, loved ones, and associates from every walk of life have gathered to pay tribute to you on this significant birthday. They have organized the event to celebrate your life as a glorious canvas of fulfillment. Before the evening is over, four individuals are going to stand and pay tribute to you and all that you have accomplished.

In this exercise, you are going to write in the voices of these four different people, each of whom will address the way you fulfilled one of your desires. In other words, you will write in the voice of the specific person who can best speak in an insightful way about how you lived in light of one of the four desires: *dharma, artha, kama,* and *moksha*.

In addition to listing your specific accomplishments, the people who pay you tribute will also talk about the things you overcame to be successful—the internal and external challenges that you had to work through to achieve all your desires, including the patterns you had to overcome that were sabotaging you from achieving your goals. They will also describe the biggest life lessons that you learned, your life philosophy and values, and the relationships and accomplishments of which you are the most proud.

In their tributes, each of the four people is going to give as many specific details as possible about what you accomplished and the glorious life you lived. As you imagine this life, you should envision it as the life you would have lived if from this day forward you were an unstoppable force, completely aligned in all your actions with your life purpose.

Why am I asking you to imagine other people providing their perceptions of you? Because in all likelihood they have perspective and are able to see things about you that you cannot, and by putting these tributes in their voices, you step into new wisdom and self-understanding that go beyond your own feelings and beliefs about yourself. And this is vital: remember, you want to access your subconscious, your heart, your intuition, not your intellect.

Again, each of the four voices is going to represent in detail how you lived in respect to one of the four desires.

One person will speak about how you succeeded in fulfilling your unique *dharma*: how, in the powerful, fulfilled future you are imagining for yourself, you have contributed to the world relative to your profession, charity work, and selfless service to others. What actions or intentions contributed the most meaning and purpose to your life? What were the specific results of following your heart? How did your life ripple out and touch and benefit the lives of others?

Another person will talk about you in the *artha* category. Specifically, what did success look like in material terms: money, home, security? He or she can talk about your health as well as any other means that were necessary for you to fulfill your unique *dharma*. (If you are a meditator, for example, the person paying tribute will talk about your meditation practice; if you're a real estate developer, he or she may detail your networking skills.)

The *kama* testimonial will address pleasure: how and in what ways your actions, thoughts, and words afforded you joy. They will describe your life in the context of beauty, enjoyment, intimacy with family and friends, how much you celebrated life, and how you tasted the sweetness of delight. *Kama* could entail sensual pleasure or the pleasure of your accomplishments; perhaps you loved playing an instrument, or reveled in long nature walks, or found your greatest joy in friendships. It will be up to your speaker to reveal to you the ways in which you were fulfilled in *kama,* the role that art, Nature, play, the things of the senses, friends, family, pets, and so on played in your life.

The fourth speaker will describe how you have lived in terms of *moksha,* your spiritual evolution. He or she will speak about the true freedom and fearlessness with which you lived, the depth of your awareness of and closeness to God or truth, how and in what ways you achieved freedom from the chains of fear, anger, grief, and anxiety as well as the comings and goings of the events of the world. This person's talk will cover how, in the larger scheme of life, you felt at peace, comfortable with yourself and your Creator or Source.

The following is an example of the four tributes that one of my students, Don, wrote in the voices of people in his life. Please note the many details included in each of Don's tributes.

Dharma Testimonial by Elizabeth Tillman,
High School Creative Writing Teacher

It's a pleasure for me to be here and to speak to you today about Don. During my many years of teaching, I have met and worked with thousands of students; however, Don stands out in my memory for many reasons. My first impression of Don was that he was the king of the passive voice—and I told him so, more than once. But after a few months in my English class for juniors he shaped up and began to turn in the best essays and reports I had read in a long time. I remember writing a note on one of his papers: "After a weekend of reading essay after essay, this is the one I was hoping to find."

Don sometimes seemed like just one more distracted kid, but as I got to know him, I realized that I was teaching a rare gem: a young man dedicated to applying his fine intellect to good ends. More specifically, he used his uncommon ability for discrimination to untangle complicated ideas and make them clear. Don was uncommonly egalitarian. There were always fascists in my classroom and plenty of bleeding-heart liberals, but it was Don who could find a thread that all could agree on and accept as common sense.

Don, even then, was drawn to trying to answer big questions. Since we didn't offer philosophy in high school, most of those questions came from his life in the Lutheran church—something for which I did not have much regard personally, but it worked for him. At least it provided fodder for thought and discussion. One of his early obsessions was the notion of righteousness. (Was it surprising he told his mom when he was twelve he wanted to be a minister?) He was drawn to that early question because of what he felt was the hypocrisy of those who claimed to be following some higher law yet violated the most basic teaching—to love one another. Love—beyond the bounds of culture and prejudice—was at his core, and he disliked greatly to see it so incompletely practiced.

It came as no surprise to me that Don chose to become a journalist and later to apply his talent and his sensibilities to writing fiction.

Some would have us believe that journalism and writing are dying professions, but that is precisely why we are desperately in need of writers like Don. Of course he was born with a talent to write. However, in each of his incarnations as a writer—as far back as eleventh grade, later as a newspaper columnist, then a short-story writer, and lastly as a successful novelist—his writing conveyed much more than just the working of a keen intellect. I feel comfortable calling Don an artist because his work consistently asked his readers to reflect upon the deeper issues and to question their own moral compass.

I was so pleased to learn Don took that early obsession with innate analytical abilities to begin inquiries into the ways we humans can more fully realize compassion in our lives. And I am just as pleased to know that I, at one time, was his teacher and that I may have played a small role in helping Don make a difference in the world through the written word.

Artha Testimonial by Alan Roberts, My Dad

I knew Don wasn't the son I expected to have when he told me he really didn't like going to the boat show. We had gone for years—it was our annual father-son activity—and we had seen hundreds of campers, tents, and boats. Who wouldn't love that? Someone not very interested in campers, tents, and boats, that's for sure.

Nor was he into cars or bicycles, except as modes of transportation. All looked the same to him. He could get just as much pleasure driving my Pontiac Catalina with a V-8 as he did in the little white four-cylinder Chevette we bought in the eighties. It didn't matter what was under the hood, and Don didn't really care to look.

Don was much the same about his possessions—carefree and a little careless.

I am proud to say that he turned that around by midlife and began to see how his attitude about these things could be detrimental. He eventually got around to remodeling his house. It took hours and hours and planning and hard work, but he turned a shack into a beautiful, energy-efficient family home—one I would be happy to live in. He did it with his own hands and hired help only when he had to. Because of this sweat, Don turned what could have been a liability into a sound investment, especially when he and Clarissa left New England.

I never imagined my son could make a living from writing, let alone save enough money for a comfortable retirement. Much to my surprise, Don managed to accumulate all the resources he and his family needed to fulfill his dreams.

After moving to Peru and renting out their house for the years they were gone, Don and Clarissa sold it for a good deal more than they'd paid. This enabled them to buy land in Minnesota for their retirement and be closer to his mom and me.

I am still amazed by the fact that so many people, including many of you, think of my son as the great writer. I just think of him as my son. So about his legacy as a writer, I'll leave that to others to decide. What I do know is that Don has always lived with a kind of balance. I don't know where he got that from—well, maybe his mother, but certainly not me. A dedicated father, husband, and not the least of all, son, he is disciplined. He never seemed to fail at being disciplined. I believe it was the thing that has enabled him to have a great career. Discipline is his key to success.

Don loves his huge garden in Minnesota, especially the apple orchard.

Thank you, son. You made me a proud father. And damn the boat show—you were always smarter than I was.

And one other thing, all kidding aside: I don't think I ever told him this before, for most of my life, I've looked up to you, son. You just seemed to know how to do it right most of the time.

Kama Testimonial by Renee Simpson, My Sister

Don's love for his family has always been first and foremost for him. Nothing seems to bring him greater joy than to spend time with his immediate and extended families. He has always found his deepest connections to himself through his family—they have been a bedrock to him, and he has always made every effort to be a meaningful part of their lives. He strove to fly to St. Louis to listen to concerts, attend weddings, baptisms, funerals. He called. He e-mailed. He was true to my adage: There is no quality time without quantity.

I am proud of my brother for the way that he has managed to overcome our familial resistance to intimacy. He's been a shining example to all of us that being vulnerable and emotionally available is not a sign of weakness and that intimacy need not culminate with a physical relationship. His way of being has had a profound effect on all those around him, not just his family. As I look around the room, I sense that if there's one thing we all have in common, it is that all of us have been inspired by having shared time with Don.

Don derived great joy in sharing his gifts, whatever he was doing. He believed and acted on the notion that authentic sharing could be just as profound as any philosophical idea.

Don and Clarissa raised two beautiful children, one adopted in Peru. They ensured that both would be bilingual, and raised them in a home filled with love.

Moksha Testimonial by Clarissa Roberts, My Wife

I always knew when Don's burden was light—he was like a gleaming star, shooting across the heavens, filling you with awe. It was just as easy to see when he was burdened by stress or regret or disappointment or frustration. He would be in a bad way, a dark place—darker than many of us would believe.

To our good fortune, Don began to recognize the fluctuations, the ups and downs, and then how to stay on the upper end of them.

This struggle led to all kinds of insights, which would serve him well as he helped others achieve a comparable liberation.

His curse turned out to be a great gift. Fortunately for him, I am infinitely patient—or nearly—and just as forgiving. And because I was so, he turned it around. And turned so many others around.

Don banished all feelings of inadequacy. He ended the cycle of regret over failure and freed himself from the self-defeating thoughts that undermine risk taking.

He also unchained himself from the desire for reassurance and encouragement, a desire that twisted the input and output of his life. He stood confident in his choices, learned to listen deeply, and acted from an authentic, intuitive place.

Step 2: The Tribute

Now that you have an overview of the foundation for this exercise, you're ready to move on to what I call the tribute part of the exercise.

In a workshop, I give people about an hour to complete their four testimonials. It may take you more time; it may take you less. I do suggest about fifteen minutes per testimonial. If it takes you more than one sitting to complete it because you don't have the time to do it all right now, that's all right. The important thing is to complete it.

During the process you may find yourself seeking comfort foods or various other distractions to avoid doing it. If you see this happening, be kind and gentle to yourself—but stick with it. Keep in mind that the exercise is a series of steps. Finish one, then when you're ready, move on to the next.

1. Choose the names of the four people who will speak about you. It's important whom you choose, so take some care with this. List the four categories on a sheet of paper: *dharma* (accomplishments, especially job or career), *artha* (material possessions and means to achieve *dharma*), *kama* (pleasure), and *moksha* (spiritual development). Under each category, list five to ten people who come to mind who could speak to that particular desire. You can list any name more than once, in as many or as few of the categories as you like.

   Although some of the names will probably be those of close friends or family, you can also choose people you've never met. For example, I had a student who wrote in the voice of C. Everett Koop, who was U.S. surgeon general at the time. She was a nurse, and she wanted him to talk about her *dharma*. She had heard Koop speak at a lecture and had listened to several speeches he had given, and she felt she could tap into his voice and that he would understand her life as a nurse in an insightful way. If you have a relative who is no longer alive but who you feel would be right to talk about one of these areas of your life, he or she could be a good choice.

   Ask yourself who knows you, your hopes and dreams, your inner truths and outer accomplishments, or who you feel would understand them if he or she did know you. Ask yourself who can speak about your potential and how you fulfilled it as well as your real purpose in the world. Who could speak well about your material, pleasurable, and spiritual capacities? Take no more than two minutes to write down names for each desire.

2. Look at your list of five to ten names for each desire and circle the name of the one person you would most like to hear from about your life relating to your fulfillment of that desire. Please pick one for each cate-

gory of desire, so you will be writing in four different voices, one per desire.

3. Now that you have the list of circled names, you're almost ready to start the process of writing testimonials. To make it easy for yourself, take four sheets of paper and at the top of each page write the name of one of the speakers and the particular desire that he or she will refer to as the context for talking about your life. Again, I recommend about an hour for completing this part of the process.

Here are some tips to help you get started:

- If you've never written in someone else's voice before—and you probably haven't—you may find yourself resisting. Think a moment. Could you imagine what your mother, father, or sibling would say in a particular circumstance? Of course you can. You could almost literally hear their voice and what they would say. It is the same for the people you have chosen to speak about you; as long as they are vivid to you and have meaning for you, you will find that you can imagine their voices, too.
- When you write in the voice of your speakers, just have the intention to be authentic, to honestly give voice to their reflection on you and the scenario of your life starting today and extending into a long future of fulfillment. If what they say is not authentic, it won't help you to uncover your Dharma Code.
- As you start to imagine what your speakers will say, although it should be ideal, it should also be practical. By practical I mean that if you aspire to be a novelist but you are forty-five and have never written a novel, can your speaker on *dharma* say, "At ninety, she has written sixty-five novels"? Probably not. Be open to inspiration, but don't allow your imagination to totally eclipse practicality. Being practical will ground your dreams in reality and make it possible for you to achieve them.
- In writing the tributes, you don't have to write complete sentences. No one is going to judge whether or not your sentence structure or spelling is perfect. You're simply going to write in a stream-of-consciousness style, noting what comes into your mind without censoring it. Write as

fast as you can. The power of this kind of writing technique is its ability to tap into your subconscious, which is where much of your deeper wisdom resides.

- To tap into it, you may need to write some words or phrases that make no sense to you. Write them down anyway. If you judge and edit what should go on the paper, it's likely you won't get to what the unconscious is trying to reveal. So don't judge; just write as the thoughts come through your mind.

- Don't worry if the first couple of sentences feel weird or if you don't get on a roll right away. Usually it takes two to four sentences for the process of writing in this new voice to begin to kick in. As long as you are committed to writing as fast as you can and not judging what's going onto the paper, and it is coming from somewhere authentic within you, it won't take you long to get the important, salient information onto the page. I've found that often after writing down something that makes no sense, you get a pearl, and if you inhibit what may seem nonsensical, your pearl won't come to the surface.

- I can't say this strongly enough: don't judge or overthink the work. The best results come when you do it spontaneously and intuitively. Do each part as fast as you can. Once you put pen to paper, don't stop writing until you're done with the tribute in that particular voice, addressing that particular desire.

It's common for people to be surprised about what winds up on the page. The point of the exercise is discovery. Allow yourself to have fun with it. Just write, and later you'll see what's on the page.

Remember, the aim of these testimonials is to discover your soul's deepest driving desire, by imagining what your life will look like after thirty, forty, or fifty years of absolutely inspired, purposeful living. So for each voice covering each desire, ask yourself: "What did I accomplish by the time the tribute celebration takes place? What were the challenges I met and moved through?

"What were the lessons I learned?

"What were the values I came away with and incorporated in my life?

"What relationships and accomplishments am I most proud of?"

Now you're ready to write a tribute in each person's voice. Make sure to complete each person's tribute, writing down all that he or she has to say about your life and that desire before moving on to the next one. Start with *dharma*, because that is the one that supports and shapes all the other desires. After *dharma*, write about *artha*, *kama*, and *moksha*, in that order.

Step 3: Drafting Your Dharma Code

Once you've completed the tributes, you are now ready to distill the information that you will use to discover your Dharma Code, the code that will describe your soul's unique reason for being. Like Laura's Dharma Code, which she later refined as "The joy in my life is this: in every moment and in every way I share all of myself," your Dharma Code will be a statement. The statement is not meant to be a shopping list of specific desires, but rather a distillation of the driving aim of what your soul aspires to. It is the desire of your *jivatman*—the life purpose with which you came into this world and that will remain a preeminent force throughout your life, constantly informing each of your four desires. Becoming aware of it, and using it to guide your life decisions in relationship to all four desires, will empower you to thrive and lead you to lasting fulfillment. That's why you are distilling these words and phrases from tributes based on your ideal scenario for your life: the words and phrases are about your best life possible, a life where from this moment onward you fulfill your full potential in every area.

This following process should take you thirty minutes or less.

1. Read through your tributes. As you do, notice which words and phrases seem to be the most compelling, the most significant. Which ones express what you feel are the key ideas and relevant themes of your life philosophy? As you read through your tributes, circle or highlight these key words and phrases.

Here are the key words and phrases that my student Don highlighted in his tributes:

applying his fine intellect to good ends . . . answer big questions . . . the notion of *righteousness* . . . the most basic teaching—to love one another . . . carefree . . . deepest connections to himself through his family . . . discipline . . . vulnerable is not a sign of weakness . . . great joy in sharing his gifts . . . a gleaming star . . . turned so many others around . . . risk taking . . . learned to listen deeply

2. Spend some time reflecting on the highlighted or circled words and phrases. The tributes, particularly these highlighted words, mark your pathway to your most compelling, most extraordinary, and fulfilled life. The words and phrases that you've highlighted are your clues to the values and priorities that will lead you to, and keep you on, that path.

   As you reflect on these key words and phrases for a fulfilled life, think about how closely your present life is in harmony with them and how far it deviates. The less harmonious your present life is with these words and phrases, the more essential it is for you to uncover your Dharma Code so that you can find your "mighty purpose."

3. Pare down your list of key words and phrases by reading over the list to yourself while considering the following questions:

   Which key words and phrases stand out or strike you as the most compelling? Which seem to include other, smaller ideas?

   Which words and phrases do you see as expressing the vital underlying themes? Which ones energize or excite you the most?

   Do any convey an idea or feeling to which you genuinely aspire?

   Circle or highlight only the key words and phrases that meet one or more of these criteria.

4. Read over the key words and phrases you've circled or highlighted, and as you begin to step into the essential ideas they convey, be aware of how your body responds. As Laura's demeanor and even her posture changed when we uncovered her soul's driving desire, you may also begin to feel lighter, inspired, or more whole as you read these words and phrases that are connected to your Dharma Code. Good feelings often unfold as we move toward a more authentic version of ourselves. On the other hand, some students have told me that the prospect of fully embodying the greatness and the qualities referred to in their list of key words and phrases can feel daunting, even scary. So as you consider them, if you notice a visceral shift one way or the other in how you feel, you have undoubtedly uncovered values and themes that are an expression of your soul.

5. Once you've pared down your key words and phrases, you're ready to draft the sentence or two or short paragraph that will be your Dharma Code. For now, write down every circled or highlighted key word and

phrase that feels like an essential part of your Dharma Code. However, keep in mind that none of these words has to appear in the final draft of your Dharma Code. They are meant to stimulate ideas and move you toward discovery. Again, you are not obligated to have them in your finished Dharma Code; your Dharma Code needs to capture the essence of them in a way that communicates to you on a deep level.

Remember, the intent of this exercise is for you to write a draft of your Dharma Code. You can always refine it later.

It is not easy or helpful to suggest any strict guidelines for what your Dharma Code should look like or how it needs to be stated. The important thing, and I cannot emphasize this point strongly enough, is that it is evocative to you, that it speaks to and motivates you. Your Dharma Code needs to be compelling to you. It must be your personal call to action. The more passion it strikes in you, the more uplifting it is, and the more you feel obliged to act whenever you think about it, the better.

In the process of drafting your Dharma Code, remember this: it has been in you all along. Throughout your life you have had glimpses of embodying it to the fullest. It was present in those moments when you felt the most alive, when you conquered your fears, when you were driven to excel, to love, to make a difference, and to courageously be your most creative and adventurous self. In other words, your Dharma Code is your essence. Because your Dharma Code is so much a part of you, it may never have occurred to you to think about it, and it may be a challenge to recognize it. The way to overcome this challenge is to consider how to put into words the essential concept that propels you to thrive and to live for the sheer joy of it. The moment you come up with the unique expression that motivates you to bring out your very best, it will be like a light going on; at that moment you will feel that you have captured, and put into words, your soul's driving force.

Here's a final thought on writing the first draft of your Dharma Code: while it is important that your Dharma Code is worded in terms that are inspiring and evocative to you, it is even more important that it be strong enough and compelling enough to move you through the doubt, fear, and obstacles you will inevitably encounter on the way to becoming and expressing your best self. Consider the following ideas for the actual wording of your Dharma Code as suggestions only.

See if you can write your Dharma Code in present rather than future tense, and in the simplest present tense form rather than the gerund form, which ends

in -ing ("I help . . ." rather than "I will help . . ." or "I am helping . . ."). It is better to state your life purpose in a positive tenor ("I have . . . ," "I am dedicated
to . . . ," "I work to . . . ," "I live as . . . ," "I honor . . . ," "I remember . . .")
rather than a negative ("I never . . . ," "I am not . . . ," "I don't . . .").

In my experience, a powerful Dharma Code must:

- Be worded in clear and practical terms (would someone you told it to understand it?)
- Be a call to act
- Be a source of guidance when you feel lost or have to choose among conflicting desires
- Guide you to meet the challenges that your tributes describe you as having walked through to achieve your ideal life (these challenges should include the dysfunctional behavior patterns that are part of your current life)

Here's the way Don phrased his Dharma Code from the key words and
phrases he extracted from his tributes: "My life and work are transformative
fire, a light in a dark world. I am disciplined, present, and persistent, always
risking so love can grow."

Here are additional examples of effective Dharma Codes written by some
of my students:

"Live creatively. Live courageously. Exercise your boundless
    capacity."
"Step into power. Express beauty and speak only the truth."
"I receive Universal, loving guidance and channel it into the world
    with faith."
"I choose love."
"I create and serve, guided only by God's fullness and my own self-
    worth."
"I discard bondage and mere survival. I lustily create my life;
    unabashedly and skillfully acting and expressing the best of who
    I am."
"I grow and create for the benefit of all."
"Contribute wholly and completely to the growth of others. Give
    purposefully and freely."

"Lead with courage, compassion, and joy."

"Listen. Expand. Create."

Keeping the qualities of an effective Dharma Code in mind, write your draft of your Dharma Code utilizing the key words and phrases from your tributes to inspire you. Don't be intimidated; have fun with it, be creative. Remember, this is just your first draft. The more you live with it and think about it, the clearer you will be about whether it communicates to you the way it's phrased now, or if it would benefit from refinement later. If it needs to be refined, ideas for phrasing it in a way that is more clear and evocative will occur to you spontaneously. Repeat it to yourself before you go to sleep and be open to any insights you may have when you wake up in the morning. The more often you say it, the more insight you will gain about any adjustments your Dharma Code might need, particularly as you start to work with the processes of relaxation and self-inquiry that will be introduced in subsequent chapters.

Step 4: Sharing Your Dharma Code

Once you have a draft of your Dharma Code, consider finding someone to whom you can read it. This can be anyone you trust who is able to listen and give you feedback in a supportive way. Often students think this automatically means the people with whom they are closest: spouses or other family members, old friends. But this is not necessarily the case. While these people know you well, the most important criterion for choosing someone to whom you can read your Dharma Code is that the person has no stake in keeping you as you are. Sometimes people who know us well want us to remain who and where we've been.

Reading your Dharma Code out loud to someone and getting his or her input on its clarity can be a powerful step to arriving at your final Dharma Code. In my workshops, I give students the opportunity to do this by pairing them with a "dharma buddy." Ideally, you can share your Dharma Code with someone who is working the *Four Desires* process, but just because someone isn't doesn't mean he or she cannot be of help. The point is to find a *dharma* buddy—or, even better, form a group of *dharma* buddies—who is like-minded and can embrace, not be threatened by, your enthusiasm and commitment to change for the better. You're looking for input, not criticism, from the person with whom you will share it.

As you move forward, please remember that, as I said to Laura, the key to allowing your Dharma Code to lead you to long-term happiness is to commit to it. This means to continue to make it burn brighter than your fears, your circumstances, and your old patterns. Knowing your purpose is only the first step; accepting it and living for it so that it guides your actions are the steps that quantitatively and qualitatively empower you to live your best life. This is such a vital part of the process of *The Four Desires* and so essential to a fulfilled life that we will return to it in the final part of the book.

> . . . .
> *Let your Dharma Code lead you, and the career and everything else your heart seeks will follow.*
> . . . .

It may also be helpful to recall Swami Rama's advice about the key to happiness. "First, become clear what your duty or purpose is in life," he said. "Second, learn to love it." Note that he broke the key to happiness into two distinct steps. Just because you recognize your soul's purpose does not mean that you will automatically love it.

I certainly experienced the disparity between getting a glimpse of my *dharma* and embracing it wholeheartedly. It took me several years of struggling with, even resisting, what appeared to be my destiny as a teacher before I embraced Swami Rama's advice. Like Rob, who wanted to be an actor and didn't realize or accept that an alternative talent of his, painting, would be the vehicle for him to fulfill his soul's purpose, I had to let go of my preconceptions about teaching yoga and about what would be an acceptable career before I recognized my *dharma* and embraced teaching as my way to fulfill it.

From the moment I began to teach, I knew that I had found something special. Teaching felt like home, far and away the most authentic way of expressing who I was and my joy of life. In this sense, nothing else had come close to giving me what teaching gave me. Yet even as I was teaching yoga and making a living from it, I wondered how or if I could make a career of something that seemed so impractical. I doubted that I even wanted to. I assumed that I should be doing and concentrating on something more practical, more grounded in day-to-day reality. Despite these judgments, I kept teaching. Thus, even though I didn't recognize it, I was following my *dharma,* and my classes grew year after year. Eventually I was able to let go of my preconceptions and see that I was fulfilling my *dharma;* not long afterward all my conflicts about teaching disappeared. At a certain point, I fell in love with it—I realized that I loved what I was doing and that I couldn't imagine doing anything else.

Life taught me, as have the lives of people whom I've taught, that by following your soul's wisdom you can create a wonderful, fulfilled life that includes earning a living doing something that you love.

As I've seen throughout the years, many of us have preconceptions about what we can and cannot do, attachments to what we should and shouldn't do. Often these preconceptions and attachments tempt us away from the counsel of our own hearts and the mighty destiny our soul longs for us to fulfill.

Few things are more powerful than learning to trust that your path to a fulfilled life—and the glorious destiny that you are meant to share with the world—is contained in your Dharma Code. This is why I say: let your Dharma Code lead you, and the career and everything else your heart seeks will follow.

CHAPTER 7

· · · ·

WATCH YOUR MIND THINK

The Key to Being Guided All the Time

You might be wondering why it should require so much effort to find or live by your soul's purpose. For the answer I turn to one of the most essential teachings of the yoga tradition, one that, I believe, is critical to achieving the two kinds of fulfillment that I discussed earlier—material and spiritual fulfillment.

The reason you have to *learn* to recognize the deeper meaning and purpose of your life is because under ordinary circumstances your mind is less than ideally suited to "hear" your soul or the subtle directives of *dharma*. Although both are ever-present and always ready to guide you, your mind needs to be trained to be able to perceive the inherent gifts of your soul as well as the guiding influence of *dharma*. The following two-minute experiment will help you understand why.

AN EXPERIMENT IN WATCHING YOUR MIND THINK

This following experiment is extremely simple: For two minutes, you are going to observe yourself thinking. For 120 seconds I'd like you to count each time you have a thought. I suggest you use a timer so you won't have to think about the time. The experiment is to simply observe your mind "think" for a period of two minutes. You might be tempted to just read past this experiment instead of doing it, but even if you didn't do the first exercise, please give yourself the experience of doing this. It will only take two minutes, and it will give you a glimpse into the way your mind works. It will also help you build a vital foundation for lasting fulfillment as well as for much of the material to come.

Make the decision to devote yourself fully to this experiment for 120 seconds. Turn off the phone. Put the book aside. Get the timer and set it for two minutes. When you are ready, close your eyes, clear your mind, and then count each individual thought that passes through your mind. Start now . . .

It's two minutes later and you've done the experiment. How many thoughts did you have? Five or six? Twenty or thirty? You might have had fewer; you might have had more. Or did you stop before the two minutes were up?

What does this experience reveal to you about your mind? The most obvious answer is that your mind is constantly moving—darting from one thought, feeling, memory, sense perception to the next. The implication of this is that most of the time you rarely perceive or genuinely experience the present. This helps explain why it's so easy to miss the guidance of *dharma* and to live without a clear sense of your soul's purpose. The point is that both the guiding intelligence of *dharma* and your essence or soul are part of a silent, sublime melody, one that is all but impossible to hear against the clatter of a busy, distracted mind. No wonder the sages of practically all spiritual traditions sought out silence. They understood that being able to tune in to infinite intelligence was vital to being guided to a supreme life.

There is another, less obvious aspect of your mind that limits its capacity to hear the wisdom of your soul or to respond to the nurturing, life-sustaining intelligence of *dharma*. In simple terms, even the most learned mind perceives only a fraction of reality. If you've ever felt like there was more to life, it's because there is.

Modern science confirms what the yoga tradition has long asserted: that our five senses—our mind's antennae—"see" what may be as little as 10 percent of the world that we live in. The result is that unless we learn how to see beyond what our eyes, ears, nose, mouth, and skin are telling us, we can never experience the totality of who we are or the world of which we are a part.

The science of meditation was developed by the ancient sages to free the mind from its normally distracted state and to make it more capable of seeing what it ordinarily doesn't see. Many of the benefits of meditation are now recognized in clinical research and widely documented, but the fact remains that until you actually experience it, it is hard to grasp just how meditation can contribute so much to the quality of your life. Until you do it, you'll have to use your imagination.

Imagine being able, at any time, to experience the joy of having ful-filled your every desire. Imagine feeling so complete that you would no longer need anyone or anything to feel 100 percent content. Imagine having insight into how to meet every challenge and accessing inspira-tion anytime you want. You can, says the yoga tradition, and that is ex-actly what is possible when you simply learn to still your mind. That is precisely what meditation is all about.

In the ultimate sense, meditation—the process of learning to still your mind—is a door to a completely different way of thinking and feel-ing. For this reason, it stands alone among all of life's endeavors because, unlike any material or intellectual pursuit, it allows you to experience the part of you that is always at peace. Meditation teaches you that you are something more than your possessions, more than your body, more than your thoughts. Indeed, the experience of meditation makes it clear that life is an infinite landscape in which you are free to shape your future ac-cording to your deepest aspirations.

Meditation eventually reveals something that is altogether too easy to forget as we go about living our lives: that life is indeed a gift and that it is indeed sacred. And if all this were not enough, meditation is one of very few things in this world that can lead you to the second kind of ful-fillment.

Meditation may be the perfect antidote for the way that most of us use our brains in the digital age. We live in a time of sensory overload and despite all our technological advances, most of us feel that we never have enough time. As a result, most of us strug-gle to fit into our day as many things as possible. This means that we are often doing more than one thing at a time—what is com-monly called multitasking. The latest research indicates, however, that trying to do two or more things at the same time may not be good for you. Multitasking has been shown to impair cognitive skills (attention, short- and long-term memory, processing speed, visual and auditory processing, logic, and reasoning). The long-term effect is that we can wind up atrophying parts of our brain and impairing its optimal functioning.

Meditation does the opposite: it moves your brain in the direction of rest and focus. Thus, learning to still your mind is not only a vital link to inspiration and an abiding sense of peace but also an incomparable method for increasing your capacity to solve real-life issues, increase insight, and help your brain assimilate all the random bits of information that it rarely has time to process. Meditation is an indispensable tool that improves memory, sharpens intellect, increases your ability to respond to stress, and even helps you process negative emotions such as grief, anger, and fear.

For all that meditation provides, it merely asks of us that we take time to do it, to simply put a few minutes aside to steady our thoughts and learn to see the beauty and wisdom that lies beyond them.

Meditation is surprisingly simple. Anyone can do it. You don't need any special training or any special gifts to reap inestimable benefits from it. You only need to be willing to practice it.

There may be no simpler and more widely practiced form of meditation than meditation on the breath. The following is a step-by-step practice that walks you through its various stages: relaxation, concentration, awareness, and finally learning to rest in the wholeness and peace that is Spirit, Soul, or Essence.

> . . . .
> *Imagine being able, at any time, to experience the joy of having fulfilled your every desire. That is exactly what is possible when you simply learn to still your mind.*
> . . . .

Before starting your meditation, you will need to prepare yourself to be guided through it. You want to be able to follow the instructions that I give you without opening your eyes to read the next instruction. Once you begin, it's vital that you move from step to step without interrupting the meditation. Here are three ways to prepare yourself to do this: you can create a recording of the instructions by reading them aloud into a cassette or digital recorder; you can purchase *The Four Desires* practice CD (www.rodstryker.com); or you can have someone you trust read the instructions to you.

If you choose to make your own recording, speak slowly and calmly. (The same should apply if you have someone else read the instructions to you.) As you read the instructions, imagine that you are leading yourself into a state of deep peace and healing. You'll notice that I've indicated in parentheses how long to wait before the next instruction. When a pause is indicated, remain silent for the specified amount of time. The Meditation on the Breath practice should take about twenty minutes.

Whether you make a recording yourself (which may involve purchasing a small recorder), arrange for someone to read the instructions, or buy *The Four Desires* CD, it requires an effort. It's important to recognize that making the effort to prepare for this meditation means that you're already engaging yourself in the process. It affirms that you're actively committed to change and to manifesting more fulfillment in your life. You should thank yourself for taking an invaluable step toward shaping your destiny.

Here are the directions for Meditation on the Breath, complete with indications of how long the speaker should wait between the stages of the process.

MEDITATION ON THE BREATH: PRACTICE

Before beginning the practice, please find a comfortable sitting position. You can either sit in a comfortable and supportive chair or in a cross-legged sitting position on a firm cushion on the floor. It is important that throughout the meditation, your body is completely at ease, therefore, if you cannot sit cross-legged for very long without becoming distracted or uncomfortable, it's preferable that you use a chair in which you can sit tall without strain. If you are using a chair, slide your lower back against the backrest, so that your spine is tall.

Adjust your posture so that the crown of your head is over the base of your spine.

(Begin recording here)

Close your eyes. Turn your attention inward and have the intention to completely relax. Be effortless. Become aware of your body. . . .

Be aware of the space that your body occupies. Now, move your awareness to the top of your head. Have the intention to completely and deeply relax the crown of your head and scalp. Be effortless. . . .

Feel your scalp, the crown of your head, deeply relax. . . .

Feel your forehead relaxing . . . your face . . . relax the back of your head . . . relax your neck . . . your throat . . . relax your shoulders . . . upper back . . . your chest or breast area . . . relax.

Feel effortlessness around your physical heart . . . feel it beating, slowly, calmly.

Relax your solar plexus . . . abdominal organs . . . lower back . . . hips. . . .

Relax your entire pelvis. . . .

Relax your legs and feet. . . .

Sense your whole body completely relaxed. Once again, be aware of your posture. Be aware that your spine is tall and have the intention to relax your whole body. Relax your whole body.

(30 seconds)

Now, bring your attention to your abdomen. Notice that as your body breathes in, your abdomen moves away from your spine. As your body breathes out, your abdomen moves toward it. Be aware of your abdomen moving on the flow of your breath. . . . Don't force or try to shape your breath. Just be aware of your abdomen and sense it move effortlessly. Be aware of your abdomen moving on the natural flow of your breath.

(1 minute)

Allow your mind to settle and to become more and more absorbed in the rhythm of your breath. Be effortless and aware of your breath by feeling your abdomen move.

(3 minutes)

Gradually notice that your breath is a perfect reflection of your mind: as your mind becomes increasingly quiet, your breath becomes more balanced, quieter, and more subtle. Continue to watch your breath.

(2 minutes)

As you continue to watch your breath, become aware of any hidden tension held in your breath, body, or mind. Wherever you sense tension, simply relax; have the intention to be completely effortless. Become more and more effortless while being aware of your body breathing.

(2 minutes)

Eventually your mind will become so quiet, so at peace, that you will experience less and less desire to breathe. Don't resist. The more relaxed your mind, the less your body will need to breathe. As your body becomes completely relaxed and your mind still, you may even experience a pause between breaths—a brief moment between the end of the exhale and the beginning of the inhale.

In this brief gap between breaths you experience a moment between thoughts. In this gap, you glimpse a timeless state of Being.

(2 minutes)

Continuing to effortlessly watch your breath, feel your breath leading you back to your Source. As you do, feel more and more at home in the gap between breaths. Just be and watch your breath. Don't try to make anything happen. The moment between breaths will unfold naturally the more you drop into complete effortlessness.

(2 minutes)

Sensing the breath rising out of and returning to a silent and infinite presence, be aware that in this moment you are whole and complete. You are a vibrant expression of infinite intelligence.

(2 minutes)

Bring your attention back to your breath. Take a few smooth, full breaths to adjust. Very slowly begin to reopen your eyes and allow your attention to come back to your surroundings.

End of practice.

This Meditation on the Breath is a simple, accessible, yet profound approach to meditation. The more you practice it, the more capable you become of stilling your mind and tuning in to *dharma*.

Now that you have at least a rough draft of your Dharma Code—your life purpose—we move to the next step of living your best life: learning how to recognize the immediate goal that your soul is inspiring you to accomplish and then learning the process for awakening your power to achieve it.

REFLECTIONS ON UPWARD-FACING DOG POSE

. . . .

Urdhva Mukha Svanasana

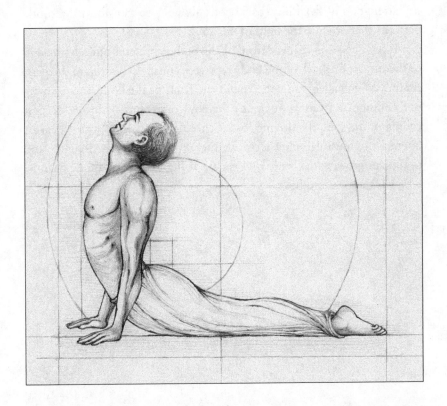

Upward-Facing Dog is a challenging and exhilarating backbend, one in which the whole body is engaged for the single purpose of opening the front torso, especially the chest—which in the yoga tradition is considered to be the abode of our spiritual heart, self-essence, or soul. Holding the pose builds strength in the legs and arms, both of which must be fully engaged, along with the abdominal muscles, to provide support for the lower back. Until we start practicing yoga, few of us spend much time bending backward; thus, consciously or unconsciously, most students will experience a degree of fear in this posture. Practically speaking, this fear relates to the concern to protect our lower back, a particularly vulnerable area of our spine. That's why it is so important that students who are new to yoga quickly learn to properly engage the muscles that support the lower back and why we should learn the principles of safe backbending before doing Upward-Facing Dog. At a deeper level, the fear that we may experience in the pose relates to confronting the often unrecognized subtle tensions that "sit" on our spiritual heart. Therein lies both the challenge and the treasure of backbending: while building physical strength and flexibility, backbends allow us to transform the subtle patterns that obscure the light of our soul.

It has been said that the front of the body represents our relationship to the future; the back of the body represents our relationship to the past. As this pose challenges us to expand the front of the body, it empowers our willingness to move forward, thereby connecting us to the deepest calling of the soul, the driving force behind all aspiration. As the heart is opened in Upward-Facing Dog, we literally feel courage, strength, and optimism grow, and a sense that we are being led to more fully become who we are meant to be.

PART III

AN INTENTION
FORMED IN
THE HEART

. . . .

CHAPTER 8

THE SCIENCE OF MANIFESTING INTENTION

Tara was overwhelmed. Her life had become an endless string of responsibilities: mother, wife, family cook, small-business owner, home-school teacher to her two children. At the same time, she remained committed to making time daily for prayer and meditation. At my workshop, she finally admitted she wanted—*needed*—help. She identified this as her critical desire, the desire that, if she could fulfill it, would positively affect everything else in her life.

After acknowledging her desperate desire for "help and clarity to manage the breakneck pace of my life," she drafted a clear and defining statement of exactly what it was that she wanted: "I achieve my goals through my work with the help of supportive partners."

Tara left the workshop focused on her resolution to get help. Suddenly, partners—people who would provide her with the help she needed to achieve her goals—began to manifest: a capable housekeeper, someone willing to step in to help with the administration of her business, a support network of other parents for home-schooling her children. This first wave of support was the easy part, but more change was needed before Tara could have what she really needed to achieve her goals.

As she tells it:

After getting this support came a tremendously painful realization—my marriage was eroding, precipitously so. It became excruciatingly

clear that my most important goal—engaging in a loving, supportive, intimate relationship that fostered a healthy family life and foundation for all other life demands—was being neglected, pushed aside,
and trampled. Several days, many boxes of tissues, and heaps of self-
recrimination later, I had a clearer understanding of my own culpa-
bility and incapacity to seek and accept help where I most needed it.

No sooner did all of this hit me when the next wave of partners
manifested, partners who would help me fulfill my most treasured
goals. My three new partners that suddenly emerged were my husband, who is committed to moving us into a new and richer relationship; a wise marriage counselor; and, surprisingly, my own self,
with a brand-new perspective.

My resolution has affected my life much, much more deeply
than I had intended, or maybe even considered possible. It has
helped me take a giant step toward fulfilling my Dharma Code,
which is "to love and be loved."

After struggling for years, Tara saw her life take a dramatic and lasting change for the better. It is now three years since she declared what she
wanted, "to achieve my goals through my work with the help of supportive partners," and she is now much further in realizing her Dharma
Code. As she tells it: "My life is filled with more amazing stuff and opportunities than I ever could have imagined."

The key to making all of this possible was getting clear about and
then acknowledging what she wanted. Tara is a living example of something Ralph Waldo Emerson is often credited with having said, "Once
you make a decision, the whole universe conspires to make it happen."

Tara changed the course of her destiny—and the destiny of her husband and her children—for the better. Doing so had everything to do
with her formulating and focusing on a resolve that was harmonious
with, and indeed an expression of, her Dharma Code, her life purpose.

"If you cling to a certain thought with dynamic will power, it finally
assumes a tangible outward form," said Paramahansa Yogananda. "When
you are able to employ your will always for constructive purposes, you
become the *controller of your destiny.*"

The place to start harnessing your power to determine your destiny
and achieve any intention is your own mind. Before Tara made her resolution, her mind was in a muddle. She knew she was dissatisfied, but she

was unclear about what she wanted, even in her marriage. The moment she made her resolve, things began to change. Tara's life illustrates a central teaching of the Vedic tradition: the most profound way to affect the course of your life is by harnessing the power of resolution or intention, which in Sanskrit is called *sankalpa*.

> . . . .
>
> *Your mind has measureless capacity to affect the quality and content of your life.*
>
> . . . .

Sankalpa is the compound of two Sanskrit words: *kalpa*, which means "a way of proceeding" or, more revealingly, "the rule to be observed above or before any other rule," and *san*, "a concept or idea formed in the heart." Thus, *sankalpa* means determination or will, an intention, conviction, vow, or, most commonly, a resolution, one that reflects your highest aspirations. In practical terms, a *sankalpa* is a declarative statement, resolution, or intention in which you vow or commit (to yourself, your teacher, a priest, or even God) to fulfill a specific goal. A *sankalpa* at first glance looks a lot like a modern-day resolution or intention.

We are all familiar with the concept of intention or resolution. It is said that the average American makes 1.8 resolutions per year. We create intentions to lose weight, find a more rewarding career, get organized, or attract the ideal relationship. We resolve to change our diet, be more disciplined, work harder, work less hard, spend more time in Nature or with our families, do something about our stress levels, enrich our spiritual life, write or read more, stop smoking, get a degree, be a greater force for good in the world, or any one of countless other things we aspire to achieve.

It's critical, however, to note that research shows that at least 80 percent of us do *not* achieve our resolutions. A recent study found that "four out of five people who make New Year's resolutions . . . will eventually break them. In fact, a third won't even make it to the end of January." Other studies have shown that the number of people who do achieve their resolutions is even smaller, perhaps as little as 8 percent. Despite all that you may have heard from motivational speakers or spiritual teachers or read in books in praise of the limitless power of intention, this statistic means that fewer than one out of ten of us achieve what we set out to achieve.

What explains this failure of at least 80 percent of us to fulfill our resolutions?

One very important reason, which I discussed at length in Part II, is that we too often focus on fulfilling our desires without giving much thought to how our desires serve the greater meaning and purpose of our lives. Another reason, from the perspective of the tantric tradition, is that there is a science to the process for manifesting intention, and if you don't apply it, you will likely end up as part of the 80 percent who don't see their resolutions fulfilled.

The simple truth is when a resolution is little more than a wish, even one that you think many times a day, it has relatively little or no impact or power to affect your destiny. However, when you work through the steps involved in achieving a resolution methodically, its reach and its power to affect your destiny become nearly limitless. Let's take a closer look at why and how.

Sankalpa or resolution holds a special and highly esteemed place in the ancient teachings. The concept of *sankalpa* appears even as early as the *Rig Veda,* the most ancient of all the Vedic texts. The art and science of applying *sankalpa* was considered to be the foundation for achieving or becoming anything of real significance.

Throughout the Vedic and tantric traditions it is made exceedingly clear that a student cannot make meaningful progress toward any worthwhile goal without first cultivating the power of resolve, what the yogic tradition calls *sankalpa shakti.* "On this path you must first awaken your *sankalpa shakti,* the power of will and determination," said Swami Rama. "Overcome your resistance. Expand your capacity. . . . you must order your body and senses to function under the leadership of your mind."

The ancient concept of *sankalpa* is predicated on the principle that your mind has measureless capacity to affect the quality and the content of your life. The ancient traditions, including the Veda, tantra, and yoga, venerated the mind and appealed to the Divine for the mind to be filled with "auspicious thoughts" because they saw the mind as the chief architect of our lives. In other words, they viewed your mind as the ruler of your fate. Accordingly, in the Vedic pantheon of gods, Indra, who represented mind at the cosmic level, was considered the chief of all the gods. "The mind is everything. What you think you become," said the Buddha.

The power to affect your future, therefore, begins by learning to focus your mind. "Each thought influences your mind and creates therein a vibration that affects your whole life, your destiny," Mani would often say. His enduring message was that to the degree you learn to collect your thoughts and then direct your mind toward an intention, there are few things that you cannot accomplish.

The tradition tells us that upon commencing any important undertaking, anything you truly aspire to achieve, your first step should be to create a *sankalpa,* a clear and definitive resolve that you *will* accomplish your goal. It is critical to recognize that there is a difference between having a desire and having a *sankalpa.* You may *want* something, but that is not the same as creating a *sankalpa* that you *will* achieve it. Consider this: a desire is little more than a feeling (sometimes strong and sometimes not so strong) related to a want—to have, to become, or to achieve—some thing; a *sankalpa,* on the other hand, is a desire that you are absolutely determined and committed *to* achieve.

A simple way of illustrating this distinction, which many parents can relate to, is the way we choose to show up for our children. Parents who understand how crucial it is that their child knows that he or she can count on them—both for the good of the child-parent relationship and for the benefit of the child's own personal

> . . . .
>
> *When a resolution is little more than a wish, even one that you think many times a day, it has relatively little or no impact or power to affect your destiny.*
>
> . . . .

development—consciously or unconsciously make a decision to follow through on promises they make to their child. If you understand this, when you make a promise to your child, you do all you can to ensure that your promise is fulfilled. You make it happen, come hell or high water. It is not always easy or convenient, but you manage to fulfill your resolve despite the challenges. At this point, your intention that your child knows that he or she can depend on you is no longer just a desire, something you would like to happen—it has become a *sankalpa,* which means that practically nothing can stop it from happening. The essential requirement is that a parent must have the desire (for example, "to show up consistently no matter what") and, concurrent with that desire, the determination that he or she *will* fulfill it. Indeed, according to the tantric tradition, this principle of marrying desire with determination is the key to making a *sankalpa* truly effective.

In practical terms, this would mean learning to get to the point where your desires and your will to accomplish them are no longer two separate things. "*Sankalpa* should be done with full determination," the

Tripura Rahasya, a sublime tantric text that includes teachings on the science for manifesting intention, tells us. When this is done, "imagination [*sankalpa*] is identical with determination." Imagine bringing this kind of resolve to your own ambitions and desires.

A *sankalpa,* by definition, focuses your mental and energetic resources and, in the process, the forces of Nature toward a specific end. Unlike a Dharma Code, a *sankalpa* is result-oriented, aimed toward fulfilling a particular goal. A *sankalpa* might focus on your intention to start a charitable organization, be a better mate and parent, fulfill a career objective, live a healthier life, resolve a health issue, deepen your spiritual practice, or complete an important project. Indeed, a *sankalpa* can focus on overcoming any challenge, including even changing the thoughts you think. It could focus on a goal as specific as buying a new house or finding the right school for your children. The only parameter of a *sankalpa* is that it needs to be authentic—something that is consistent with the deeper meaning and purpose of your life. In other words, your *sankalpa* must be in harmony with—and ultimately serve—your Dharma Code.

By the time you finish applying the methodologies in this part of the book, you will have specified a desire, based on your soul's purpose, that you intend to achieve in the next six to eighteen months—a time frame that will allow you to focus your attention and capacities on achieving something meaningful, a desire that is truly in the service of your soul's purpose.

The Science Behind the Power of the Mind

Do you recall the first time you discovered the power of a magnifying glass to concentrate the sun's rays? I do, and I definitely remember that it can be a powerful and dangerous thing in the hands of an unsupervised eight-year-old boy. The power of the magnifying glass comes from the way the glass is shaped, which allows it to focus and thereby intensify what is normally diffused sunlight. We can draw a parallel between the ability of a magnifying glass to affect sunlight and the power of a *sankalpa* to affect your destiny.

As we've seen, under normal conditions your mind and its thoughts are diffused. The power of resolve focuses and concentrates your thoughts and thereby increases your mind's capacities. Through that process, your mind's potential is magnified. This is common sense when you think about it. Those whose thoughts are most unified around an idea or intention, regardless of their field of endeavor, are the ones who invariably accomplish the most. "Nibbling is useless. He alone who becomes mad with an idea sees the light," Mani would often say.

Sankalpa, resolve, or intention creates a focal point that awakens the latent power of the mind and allows it to become significantly more capable. When it is applied methodically, *sankalpa* empowers the mind to lead us to new heights, ones to which an unfocused mind, one that lacks resolve, is simply incapable of leading us.

Resolution also increases our capacity to discern and thus to take the specific actions necessary to manifest the results we desire. Conversely, when the mind is less than completely unified around a resolution, it is far less directed and effective and therefore less capable of achieving its intentions. As the Bhagavad Gita describes it: "For those who lack resolution [*sankalpa*], the decisions of life are many-branched and endless."

In recent years, theories about the power of intention to influence the world around us and to attain or attract the object of our desires have become more widely accepted. In part, this is because more of us are discovering for ourselves that intention or resolve attracts our desired aims or helps us to achieve them. Recent scientific research is helping to prove that our intentions have the power to affect the future. And who doesn't want to believe that?

The understanding of the mind's capacity to affect the material world has been part of Western science for a long time. The concept of the placebo effect, which was first discussed about three centuries ago, refers to the principle that people who are sick can get better if they believe the doctor has given them something that will help them, even though, in reality, they are taking something that has no therapeutic value. Scientists researching the placebo effect consistently find that 30 to 35 percent of people who are given a placebo do get better. In other words, approximately a third of the people suffering from an illness get better simply because their minds believe that they should be getting better.

The power of the mind's role to affect our health and well-being is also reflected in the finding that a doctor's belief in the value of a treatment can affect his or her behavior, and thus what his or her patient believes. Indeed, research shows that people get better at a higher rate when they are being treated by someone who they perceive truly believes in the medication or the procedure that is being given to the patient. Yes, the mind can and does affect our body and our health.

Research is also demonstrating the mind's capacity to affect things other than our own body. A recent study that forced skeptics in the scientific community to take notice of the mind's potential to affect material changes outside of one's own body was reported in *The New York Times.*

Researchers at Columbia University announced their rather startling finding that women in a fertility clinic were almost twice as likely to get pregnant when, unknown to them, total strangers were praying for their success. The clinic was in Korea, and the praying strangers were members of various Christian denominations in the United States, Canada and Australia. They were given pictures of the patients for whose pregnancy they were entreating God, but no other identifying information. Women in the prayed-for group had a pregnancy rate of about 50 percent, versus 26 percent for women in the control group. The Columbia researchers expressed surprise at the magnitude of this difference, saying that they did not expect to find any benefit to prayer at all. . . .

What makes the Columbia study so mystifying is that neither the patients nor the staff members at the fertility clinic were even aware of its existence. So the apparent influence of prayer could not be attributed to their beliefs or expectations or to some kind of placebo effect.

The cutting edge of scientific exploration is helping to unveil a new understanding of the power of intention. We are just at the beginning of a new frontier that is taking shape at the intersection of sciences such as quantum physics and the ancient esoteric teachings. Thanks to a growing body of research, we find ourselves at a new frontier where Western analytical thought is starting to unveil the mystery of where and how the hidden world of thought meets the world that you and I touch, taste, smell, hear, and see. Pioneers in fields such as epigenetics, which includes the study of the mind's effects on our genes, and psychoneuroimmunology, which studies the interaction between psychological processes and the nervous and immune systems, are helping to validate the assertions of the ancient teachings about how, when properly focused, the mind has the capacity to affect matter—the nonmaterial can and does affect the material.

CHAPTER 9

. . . .

WHAT IS A RIGHT DESIRE?

I've worked with people who have successfully applied *sankalpa* to achieve everything from solving family conflicts to healing a life-threatening illness, starting a spiritual practice, funding a charitable organization, overcoming fertility issues, developing new talents, breaking old habits, and reducing the debilitating effects of chemotherapy. Others have used *sankalpa* to find their dream job, increase their income, attract a compatible mate, sell their home in a depressed real estate market, and, in several cases, publish the book they were writing. Others who, feeling that they had every material thing they could want, used *sankalpa* to change how they saw themselves or their world and to manifest a humanitarian project. Each person's experience—and I will share a number of these stories in the pages that follow—illustrates the extraordinary power of the methodical use of *sankalpa*.

At this point, you now have at least a first draft of your Dharma Code, which means that you are armed with a principle to guide as well as empower you to navigate your life according to your soul's design. The next step will be to find exactly how your Higher Self or soul intends to manifest that purpose in

. . . .

The vows we make, whether constructive or destructive, whether made consciously or unconsciously, are the forces that create our world, our destiny.

. . . .

the near future. To do this, we will turn our attention to unveiling the specific desire or goal—your *sankalpa*—that your heart truly wants you to fulfill in the next six to eighteen months.

Now comes the critical question: how do you identify the specific desire that would best serve your Dharma Code? In other words, what specifically, if you could achieve it in the next six to eighteen months, would enrich your whole life and, in the process, contribute to fulfilling the meaning and purpose of your life?

At first glance, the answer might seem obvious. If you're financially strapped, wouldn't you just create a *sankalpa* to make more money at your current job, find a better-paying one, or win the lottery—in other words, a *sankalpa* that focuses on achieving a desire in the realm of *artha* (finances and material security)? Not necessarily. When it comes to desires, the obvious answer isn't always the right one. That's because until you learn otherwise, the obvious answer almost always comes from your intellect, and your intellect isn't completely capable of knowing which intention will best serve you. Your soul, however, has a way of always knowing what you need to serve your higher purpose and, at the same time, what your next best step should be in order to experience the lasting happiness you seek.

The point is, we all know, more or less, what we *want*; we don't always know what we *need*. Victoria's story is a powerful example of just how true this can be.

Victoria's Experience

Victoria was in her mid-fifties when she was told she would never again walk without a cane or crutches. A few days earlier, she had been hit by a car, which broke her hip and several ribs and crushed the bones in one of her legs. I happened to see her shortly after her surgery and the initial prognosis from her doctor.

Victoria had, in the past, worked with the process of *The Four Desires* and fulfilled several *sankalpas,* including successfully creating and navigating a challenging career transition. Her intention now was to use her power of resolve to help herself heal. Unwilling to accept the doctor's prognosis, she assumed, quite logically, that her *sankalpa* should focus on *artha*—which entails health and well-being. Her goal was to learn to walk comfortably again, resume playing golf, and even dance. Thus, her *sankalpa* was, "I can walk and am completely healed from my physical injuries." In combination with her *sankalpa*, I suggested to Victoria that she use specific vital relaxation techniques that empower *sankalpa*, in addition to visualization and meditation (processes that I will walk you through in Part IV).

A month or so later, Victoria and I spoke. That was how I learned that the work she was doing was not having the effect on her body that she had hoped for. She told me that she had made no progress since we had seen each other. I was tempted to ask her to be patient, but stopped short when she acknowledged something that her relaxation practice had revealed: being completely dependent on those around her had forced her to see something that until now she had been unwilling to admit, which was that her boyfriend of fourteen years had long been distant and unsupportive, and now that she really needed him, he was more distant and less nurturing than ever.

Despite being "together" with him, Victoria had felt alone for a long time. She realized that she needed to heal more than her body; it was time to heal her relationship with relationship. Victoria recognized that she needed to focus her attention on fulfillment of *kama*, the second desire, which relates to love, closeness, intimacy, and relationship. The more we spoke, the more obvious it seemed that Victoria's first step to healing was less about her body and more about her heart.

If she was going to heal, she needed to address her fear of being alone. If she was going to walk again, she had to be strong enough to "walk away" from a less-than-nurturing relationship. I helped her craft a new *sankalpa*. Her resolve would no longer be "I am completely healed from physical injuries." Her new resolve became "I feel loved. I stand, walk, and dance happily on my own, surrounded only by people who care for me."

From the moment she refocused her *sankalpa*, Victoria's physical healing accelerated. Almost instantly, she felt different. She was now inspired and uplifted; most important, she was now prepared to face the physical challenge of learning to walk again and stand completely on her own. Less than two years later, much to the doctor's surprise, Victoria not only stands without a cane but walks (practically skips most of the time), plays golf, and practices and teaches yoga. Her former boyfriend is no longer part of her life. Victoria is proof that when you collect your resolve, commit all of your resources, and direct them properly, you can create real, lasting, and meaningful change.

It's important to understand that, unlike with a Dharma Code, you will have many *sankalpas* over the course of your life. *Sankalpas* change because your needs evolve and also because your soul is engaged in helping you increase your capacity to meet your life's circumstances. In other words, as you and your needs change, so will your *sankalpas.* Therefore, after fulfilling a particular *sankalpa,* you will want to harness your mind's capacity to shape your destiny by determining the next specific goal or intention that will best serve your *dharma.* For example, not long after Victoria healed her broken leg, she created a *sankalpa* that focused on her spiritual life or *moksha.* Her goal was to ensure that meditation and prayer played a larger and more prominent role in her life.

Choosing Your *Best* Desire

To answer the question of how to choose the "right" desire, consider Matthew 6.33 from the Christian New Testament: "Enter the kingdom of Heaven and righteousness and all things shall be added on to thee." The Vedic scriptural source *Chandogya Upanishad* conveys the exact same principle this way: "His desires are right desires, and his desires are fulfilled." The terms *righteousness* and *right desires* point us back to the fact that the right desires are those that are in line with our higher purpose. The Sanskrit term for such desires is *satyakama,* which means "true desire." The will to act upon such desires is called *satyasankalpa,* or "true resolve."

How do you find your *satyakama,* your true desire? The answer is to ask your soul. Steeped in soul, you no longer have to try to distinguish "thy" will from "my" will; soul is where universal will and individual desire merge. As Lord Krishna states in the Bhagavad Gita, "I am desire itself, if that desire is in harmony with the purpose of life."

If you have little or no meditation experience, you might assume that soul is accessible only to those few who have dedicated their lives to finding and experiencing it. The good news is that this is not the case. As the *Yoga Vasistha* makes clear, "This self is neither far nor near. It is not inaccessible nor is it in distant places: it is what in oneself appears to be the experience of bliss, and is therefore realized in oneself." In other words, anytime you experience profound happiness or bliss in your life you are actually experiencing your soul. You may not know it, but the joy you are feeling is coming from you. It *is* you. The key is to learn to be able to access it whenever you want. That is where the practice of meditation comes in.

The process of meditation teaches that experiencing your soul is neither complicated nor difficult, but, as we saw earlier, it does require that you do it.

"I'd love to meditate. I'm sure it would do me a lot of good, if only I had the time, but I barely have enough time to do the things that need to get done. Maybe one day . . ." I've heard similar comments countless times. Time—or more to the point, a lack of it—is the reason many people give for why they don't learn to meditate, or, if they have meditated in the past, why they are unable to sustain a regular practice.

The majority of us do struggle with time. We feel the constant pressure to balance working or looking for work or being a full-time parent with making time for family and friends, ensuring that we eat properly, that we get exercise, and that all the bills are paid, not to mention having to cope with life's unexpected challenges. No wonder many people feel that from a practical perspective, they can't afford to take time away from their busy lives to meditate. The odd thing is that when we understand what meditation gives us, we realize that the opposite is true: we can't afford *not* to meditate.

We may be busier than ever, but look around—we are not necessarily happier. Life today is full of modern conveniences and technological wonders; it is packed with responsibilities and obligations, but where do you go to consistently find the joy and clarity that allow you to make sense of it all and to enjoy life to the fullest? Peace of mind is—and always will be—the answer to this vital question. Peace of mind is one of life's most precious treasures because it is the one thing that allows you to feel at home, both within yourself and in the world, no matter your circumstances. Taking a few minutes to step away from your activities and meditate is the simplest way to ensure that your life is as rewarding and meaningful as it is busy. Meditation is not just for those who are looking to prosper spiritually—it is for everyone who wants to get the most out of his or her life.

"Five to ten minutes a day of meditation—that's all it takes to ensure that you are beginning to meet your need for peace." This is what I tell people who say that they don't have the time to meditate. If they tell me that they can't find even five to ten minutes, my response is, "If you really can't find even just a few minutes to do the one thing that can ensure you will enjoy life to the fullest, maybe it's time to consider the life you've created for yourself." As you read this, if you are still doubting whether taking a few minutes out of your busy life is worth it, remember this adage: without peace of mind there is no such thing as lasting happiness.

The first step to experiencing your soul is learning to still your mind, as you did with the Meditation on the Breath in Part II. It's possible for anyone, in a single meditation session, to get at least a glimpse of stillness—and of a unique kind of contentment, the contentment that is your soul's nature. Your soul, inherently aligned with *dharma* in the largest sense, is and will always be complete and content.

When your desires are inspired by your soul, they are the means by which your short-term goals in any of the four categories of desire become the way you manifest your soul's overriding purpose or *dharma*.

So the question you will want your soul to answer is something like this: "Given my present circumstances, which one of the four desires contains the goal that you, my soul, would have me achieve or pursue next?"

What You Really Want May Surprise You

At the start of my Yoga of Fulfillment course, I ask participants to let go of their expectations and to forget everything they *thought* they wanted out of the course. I then ask them to take a moment to imagine being completely content, to conjure the feelings that they would have if they already had everything they wanted—in other words, to imagine needing no person or thing to feel whole and complete. After a moment, I then pose the following question: "If you were consistently this content—if you could permanently abide in this feeling—would your goals or wants *change?*" The room becomes quiet as participants consider what it would be like to let an abiding sense of peace and contentment guide all of their future choices. An instant later, I get the answer: for the majority of them—and for most of us—the answer is, "Yes, my goals or wants would change."

This is because, as we've seen, the simple yet often confusing truth is that while most of us know what we want, we don't always know what we need. As the ancient teachings tell it, wants are typically related

> . . . .
> *Soul is where universal will and individual desire merge.*
> . . . .

to the desire for things that are pleasant (*preya* in Sanskrit) and are generally born from our conditioning or from our base impulses. On the other hand, needs are desires that are related to the intrinsic desires of the soul (*shreya*) to fulfill its higher purpose. Thus, to the degree that you are able to access your soul and allow it to guide you, the less compelled you are to act on desires born from fear, old patterns, low self-esteem, and past hurts.

To listen and be able to hear or see what your soul would have you be, become, or achieve, you have to be able to at least approach a state in which your mind is still, so that you can rest and see your soul's inherent state of wisdom (*prajna*) and compassion (*karuna*). When you do this, the soul guides you in a way that your intellect never could. Randy's story is a very practical illustration of this.

Randy's Story

Randy was very clear about what she wanted. She was a doctoral candidate in clinical psychology and she wanted to finish her dissertation. As she explained it:

> I was on an extended "working vacation" when I attended the Yoga of Fulfillment. I had been procrastinating on my final step: finishing my dissertation. I was also preparing to begin an intensive clinical position working ridiculous hours with severely mentally ill children. To understand the significance of what I accomplished thanks to *The Four Desires,* I think it's best that you have some background.
>
> I am very good at taking care of myself when I am on vacation, even a working vacation; however, during times of high stress, I am

pretty brutal to myself. I have a tendency to skip meals, deny myself water and sleep, and be extremely self-critical when all of my work is not complete. Ironically, I would never advise anyone else to treat him- or herself in a similar way. For many years those behaviors fueled me and I accomplished quite a bit but with very little enjoyment. My only relief was when a task was complete.

In your workshop, during the Bliss Meditation that you walked us through to help us identify which of the four desires we needed to address, I had an insight. I saw that my procrastination had more to do with a kind of fragmentation than a lack of self-discipline. I realized that I had a spiritual self and a professional self and the two were strangers. That fragmentation was paralyzing me, thus I was getting nothing done and was increasingly hard on myself.

That helped me make a critical decision: rather than mercilessly willing myself into getting the dissertation done at all costs, I committed to take care of myself throughout the process—if and when I finished it, it would come out of an embrace of my whole self. So instead of focusing on the first of the four desires, *dharma,* I saw that I needed to nurture *artha*—in other words, to honor the means that would allow me to achieve the end I was seeking.

I left the workshop with a resolve that surprised me. Instead of creating a *sankalpa* like "My dissertation is finished" or something that related purely to accomplishing a work objective, I decided to express my commitment for a short-term goal in very different terms, ones that for me were very counterintuitive: "I express all of myself through self-nurturing acts." I left the workshop carrying that sentence in my pocket and I repeated it many times throughout the day.

A few weeks after the workshop, my new position began and I had not worked on my dissertation in a month. I promised myself I would not work on it until I felt moved, not bullied into doing so. I repeated my new resolve daily, when I prepared my meals, when I went for walks, when I took five minutes in between clients to sit quietly.

A few weeks into my new position at the clinic, the logical part of me began thinking that I should trade in my resolution to nurture myself—I needed to return to my old way of doing things or the dissertation was never going to get done. But something told me to hang on just a little longer.

A few days later, an idea popped into my head about my project, and I quickly wrote it down on a scrap of paper. The next day I went to my computer, dusted off my data set, and for the first time in two years I was excited about my dissertation. Two weeks later, I handed in a completed draft. Most important, I felt rested, invigorated, and well-nourished . . . and pretty freaking happy!

By concentrating on what she actually needed—nurturing herself—Randy was also able to finish her dissertation. And because she focused on nurturing herself, she found joy in the process, and for the first time she did the work with much less cost to her health and spirit. In addition, her writing came more easily and quickly than it had before. The fact that she achieved more than just a finished dissertation was no accident. It was the result of the deliberate and systematic approach of formulating and working with her *sankalpa*. She walked through a process—the same one that I will lead you through—whereby she first identified the specific "thing" she needed and then applied the right tools to get it. Randy got precisely what she asked for—and more. And so can you.

CHAPTER 10

. . . .

THE *SANKALPA* EXERCISE

The process of drafting your *sankalpa* is a seven-step process. I've broken the process down systematically to ensure that by the time you have completed all of the steps you will have a powerful and effective *sankalpa,* one that is truly unique and authentic to you. Even if you think you already know what you want, I strongly recommend that you go through the entire process. I guarantee that at the very least, it will reveal to you one or two things about your desire of which you would otherwise be unaware. And I also guarantee that the process will be engaging as well as revealing.

I suggest that you read the entire process before launching into the first step. Seeing how each step leads into the next, prior to actually starting the process, provides you with a sense of clarity and momentum that will help you craft a *sankalpa* and increase the likelihood that you will achieve it. The process, you will soon see, begins with a guided meditation. The Bliss Meditation will prepare you to identify the unique desire that you intend to achieve in keeping with your soul's purpose in the next six to eighteen months. As it did for Victoria and Randy, whose stories you just read, the meditation may make you aware that the desire you need to fulfill is different from the desire you currently believe is the right one. Since the Bliss Meditation is a guided meditation, either you will need to create a recording of the instructions or you can purchase my recording of it at www.rodstryker.com. You will also need the book in reach as well as a pen or pencil and several sheets of paper to complete the exercise.

The Big Picture

The first step of this process is to review the four desires. Don't worry if you don't remember them in detail now. I'll list them again for you and provide a brief description of each in the instructions for the exercise. They will play a crucial role in the process of identifying the one desire on which you will base your resolution, your *sankalpa*.

The second step is the Bliss Meditation, which will lead you to experience the complete contentment of your soul as well as activate a profound state of healing and vitality. In this state, you will be able to access your intuition, the wisdom of your inner teacher, or Higher Self.

The third and fourth steps guide you to your soul's wisdom, which will direct you to one of the four desires—the one that you need to fulfill.

The fifth step will help you access your intuition to make a list of the ways fulfillment in that category would touch and affect your life for the better.

The sixth step is to determine the specific goal or intention that your soul is prompting you to achieve.

The seventh step will guide you to write the first draft of your *sankalpa*.

THE *SANKALPA* EXERCISE

Step 1

Below is a list of the four desires with a description of each. Read the list to become more familiar with the four desires, and keep this book close by. When you complete the Bliss Meditation (Step 2), you will need to have the book open to the page with this list so that you can open your eyes and immediately refer to it.

As you read through the four desires now, it's important not to anticipate which one of them your soul might choose as its priority. Don't try to figure anything out ahead of time. In order to move through this process intuitively, it's critical that after reviewing the four desires, you continue the process and do the Bliss Meditation as your next step.

Dharma. The first desire is the longing for purpose, the drive to become who you are meant to be. This desire is the longing to fulfill your potential and contribute to the world. As described earlier, *dharma* revolves around the understanding that the world and all beings in it are linked. Thus, *dharma* is the longing to support the larger good. In specific terms, *dharma* focuses on how you embody virtue in your day-to-day life. This refers to your career as well as your other roles in the world provided that they give you a sense of contributing to something greater than your own personal needs. *Dharma* can include your job or being a full-time mom, environmentalist, Scout leader, or PTA volunteer. The aim of *dharma* is for a fulfilled life that is balanced and sustainable and that positively reflects the deeper meaning and purpose of your life. It speaks to the drive for selflessness, charity, and being a living example to yourself and others of what you truly aspire to be and become.

Artha. The second desire is the longing for the means you require to fulfill your *dharma* and also to tend to the other two desires. It includes the desire for financial and material security, physical well-being, and a stable, secure home. It also includes any other means that support you in the pursuit of your higher ideals and goals.

Kama. The third desire is the longing for pleasure: sensual pleasure, sexual pleasure, friendship, intimacy, family, beauty, art, fellowship, play, adventure, creativity, or joy. It also includes the desire for the pleasure that accompanies ambitions fulfilled (all things first aspired to and then achieved produce a feeling of pleasure).

Moksha. The fourth and final desire is the longing for true freedom and spiritual awareness. This means being able to live fully, unburdened by your life and the things in it. *Moksha* is the intrinsic desire to realize a state beyond the confines of the other three desires. It is the longing to move beyond all suffering and fear and realize the highest of all joys. It is the hunger to know and merge with the highest Truth, Essence, or Creator.

Step 2

Now that you've refreshed your memory about the definitions of the four desires, you are ready to begin the Bliss Meditation, a meditation designed to open the door to constructing your *sankalpa* from an absolutely intuitive and creative place. I've designed it to take you to that source. When you meditate, remember to have the book next to you, open to the list of the four desires so that you can refer to it in Step 4, when the directions instruct you to open your eyes. However, it's important that your eyes are closed throughout the Bliss Meditation practice—do not open them until it is indicated in Step 4.

THE BLISS MEDITATION PRACTICE

Sit tall, either in a comfortable and supportive chair or in a cross-legged sitting position on the floor. Keep the book open to the list of the four desires by your side.

(Instructions begin here)

Close your eyes. Become aware of your body. . . .

Just relax and feel your body at rest. . . .

Become aware of effortless breathing. . . . Feel the whole body and feel it breathing effortlessly. . . .

(1 minute)

Begin to count backward on your breath. Start at the number ten. Whenever you notice your body breathe out, go backward one count. First exhale, nine; next exhale, eight . . . Each breath is a step backward, where you feel your body and mind relax more and more deeply . . . continue . . .

The closer you get to zero, the more your body and mind approach a state of complete ease. . . . On each exhale, peel away another layer of stress and tension. . . .

(Pause)

At zero, rest in complete stillness and peace. For a moment, just feel the presence of stillness and peace.

(1 minute)

Now, bring your attention to your forehead in the space between your eyebrows . . . as you hold your attention there.

(1 minute)

Become aware of your body breathing.

Don't force or try to shape your breath . . . just be aware of the point between your eyebrows and your body breathing . . . the more effortless you can be, the better. . . .

(1 minute)

Allow your awareness to connect your breath to the point between your eyebrows. Now, when you notice the body breathing in, your awareness moves from the point between your eyebrows to the midbrain, which is sometimes called the third eye. The midbrain is a point in the middle of your brain, roughly between your temples. When you notice your body breathing out, sense your awareness moving from that point back to the point between your eyebrows . . . continue. Just continue to feel your awareness move from one point to another on the movement of your breath. . . .

As you breathe in, awareness moves from the center of the eyebrows to the midbrain, as you breathe out, awareness moves from the midbrain to the eyebrow center.

(2–3 minutes)

As your mind begins to settle, you will begin to feel the practice becoming more effortless and a growing sense of calm. Continue. . . .

(2 minutes)

Gradually, you will become so relaxed, your mind so quiet, that you will be able to rest, your whole being absorbed in a rhythm of deep rest and contentment.

(2 minutes)

When you experience this, sense yourself becoming fully absorbed in this center. Just be there. Watch, feel, and listen.

(2 minutes)

As the mind and body enter into a rhythm of deep peace and effortlessness, you begin to sense that your awareness, at the point between your eyebrows, moves in and out on its own, independent of the breath. Eventually, you can stop thinking about and working with the breath and just be aware of a kind of effortless pulse, moving in and out of the third-eye center.

Gradually feel a sense of bliss unfolding, your whole being flooded with a boundless sense of contentment and joy. Don't try. Just be aware and, at the same time, completely effortless. Contentment will continue to unfold the more completely you let go into effortlessness.

(2 minutes)

Now become aware that the *source* of this contentment and joy you are experiencing is actually coming from you. It is you. Continue letting go into the meditation until you feel that *you* are the source of joy and bliss.

Eventually your body will feel so full of ease that you won't need to do the practice anymore. At that point, notice a feeling of deep peace both inside and outside you.

Remain in this place for as long as you like. The meditation is complete. Whenever you're ready, you can move to the next step.

Step 3

With eyes closed, tune to your wisdom center—the place of knowingness within you. For many people, it's in the gut. For others, it may either be in their heart or third-eye center. The important thing is to just settle and tune in to a feeling of knowingness and certainty within you. Resting in a deep state of contentment, experience the part of you that knows exactly what you need and what you don't need. Feel connected to the inner core of truth that is always ready and fully capable of guiding you to your best life.

Step 4

Now, slowly open your eyes and gaze at the description of the four desires in the book you have open next to you. Continue to rest in contentment, and pose the following question to your Higher Self. Calmly ask: "Which one of the four desires, if it was fulfilled in the next six to eighteen months, would best serve my highest purpose or *dharma*?"

The instant you pose this question, allow your inner voice to provide you with an answer that pinpoints the particular desire that will best serve your highest purpose. The response from your soul will be decisive and clear. If you received a clear and definite answer, great. If not, or if confusion has slipped in, it's because your rational mind is either blocking or doubting your inner voice.

If this occurs, retrace your steps. The good news is that it won't take as long this time. Close your eyes. Repeat the meditation technique, linking the effortless flow of the breath with the movement of awareness at your third eye. Then follow the steps I've described that lead up to posing the question. The moment before you ask the question again, make sure that you are experiencing the knowingness within you. It is there. Relax and you will feel it.

Once you pose the question, be open to either a sensation or an inner voice, or, as you look at the page in the book that lists the four desires, notice which one draws your attention. It may feel more positive than any of the others, appear brighter, or stand out from the other three in some other way. The important thing is to stay out of your intellect. Don't let your rational mind take over this process; it must be organic and intuitive.

As soon as you have a clear idea of the specific category of desire to which your intuition has pointed, circle it or make note of it.

Step 5

You're now going to get specific about a goal within the category of desire that your intuition has chosen by using a simple but amazing methodology called Mind Mapping. This system was first developed by neuroscientist Tony Buzan, who, while developing a strategy to tap into the potential of the brain, came up with the concepts of Radiant Thinking and Mind Mapping. The beauty of Mind Mapping is that it takes almost no time to learn and yet allows you to expand your creativity and your access to your intuition exponentially.

To start Mind Mapping, you will need a blank sheet of paper. Start by drawing an oval or circle approximately two inches wide in the middle of the page. In the middle of the circle, write the name of the desire category that came up in your meditation. If your desire was *artha*, your circle will begin as below.

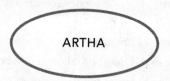

You are now going to make a list, an inventory of what fulfillment in that category might touch or affect you for the better, but first you have to let go of all your preconceptions. This list will be an inventory of what fulfillment in that category might touch or affect for the better. Here's an example of a list written by Eric, a participant in a Yoga of Fulfillment workshop I recently taught, who came to the seminar longing for some kind of change, both in his career and in his relationship to his children. The desire that his intuition had pointed him toward was *artha*. However, fulfilling *artha* is a very general concept. To gain a clearer understanding of what his *sankalpa* should focus on, he needed some additional insight. When Eric made his list, his intuition spontaneously provided him with the following details related to this desire: *money, choice, home, car, peace, joy, vacation, time, rest, creativity,* and *kids' education.* Many of these ideas surprised him. For instance, Eric never thought that fulfilling his means would be tied to creativity, time, or, for that matter, rest. And that's exactly why I'm having you create your own list in this particular way. The point is to create an opportunity for discovery.

Let's take a look at how Eric found his associated words.

After writing the word *artha* and drawing a circle around it, Eric drew a single line extending from the circle:

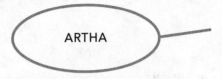

Next, Eric wrote on this line the first word or concept (two or a maximum of three words) that came into his mind associated to the fulfillment of that desire. He didn't think or judge what he heard; he just sensed what he spontaneously associated with the desire that was in the center of the circle (remember your word may be different). Eric heard the word *choice*, so he wrote it down on the line extending from the circle:

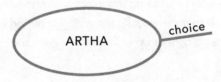

Eric then drew another line extending from the circle. Instantly another idea popped into his mind, *home*, which he wrote down on this line:

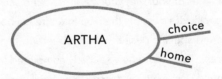

Continuing the process and writing as quickly as he could, he drew another line and jotted down the first word or concept that came to mind. He kept going until he had surrounded his circle with extended lines and the words he associated with *artha*. The eleven words his unconscious associated with this category of desire gave him a unique sense of what it would mean to him to have his desire for *artha* fulfilled.

Now it's your turn. Take no more than one minute to jot down all the words your subconscious associates with the desire that your intuition has selected to be in the middle of the circle. Don't try to take a shortcut. Do it exactly as Eric did. Start with writing down the desire and drawing the circle around it, and then draw one line at a time with its associated word before drawing the next line. Be sure to write down ten to twelve associated words so that you will start to develop a vision of what your intuition is telling you about your desire. Be prepared for your intuition to reveal aspects of your desires you may not have thought about. It is vital to do this exercise as fast as you can. Don't be careless, just fast. Remember you are not calling or relying on your intellect for answers. There is no right or wrong, and this is not a test!

Step 6

Once you've finished your Mind Map, it's time to start to shape the particular goal or intention that your soul is prompting you to achieve. Remember, unlike your Dharma Code, which is a statement of general principle that applies universally to all areas of your life, your desire and the *sankalpa* that will define it need to be specific. It's possible that you may already be ahead of me and have intuited what the specific desire is that you intend to fulfill in the next six to eighteen months. The steps you've already completed may have rekindled and intensified an old desire, or the process may have uncovered an intention that until now you hadn't given any thought. Or perhaps at this point you know the category of desire and the ideas your soul associates to it, but you haven't yet identified exactly how to phrase the precise goal that will be the basis of your *sankalpa*. The next step is to distill all your associated words and specify the specific intention your soul wishes to fulfill.

Eric, after surveying his list of words associated with *artha*, realized that all the steps of the process were pointing to one thing: selling his business.

What do your associated words tell you? What specific goal are they pointing you toward? Consider the larger scheme of your life and be mindful of any intuitive feelings so that you can discern the exact desire your soul wants you to fulfill.

Once your specific goal is clear to you, write a short description of a scene that depicts you having accomplished your desire. The description should be two or three paragraphs and should take no more than ten minutes to write. Allow your imagination and inspiration free rein to describe in detail what you want to achieve or become. Remember to focus your description on the one category of desire that you have been led to and, if you like, revisit the inventory of associated words in the diagram to give you more information.

As you write about your desire being fulfilled, be aware of the feelings that arise. Notice that the more specific and real your desire becomes as you envision fulfilling it, different emotions, such as enthusiasm, excitement, and even delight, may start to bubble up. This is a positive sign, and it is important that you include these emotions in your description of what it would be like to have your desire manifested. Be sure to include in the finished version any palpable sense of victory, joy, love, or celebration that you experience with the fulfillment of your desire.

In other words, if the desire that came up for you is *dharma* and you are writing about what it will be like to get the job of your dreams, don't just write about what the job entails, the place where you work, and who you work with; also include the feelings that accompany your experience of the job.

Having an emotional association with materializing what you want is vital and plays a crucial role in empowering your *sankalpa* (which you are almost ready to write). Invoking feelings in combination with your resolution is critical to your resolution being powerful enough to bear fruit.

Here is the scene Eric described:

For my wife and me, selling our business was the start of a new life. With the money it provided, we took six months off. We spent an ideal summer. The kids had the time of their lives. For the first time in as long as I can remember, I know what it feels like not to be chained to financial stress and whether or not we could pay bills or run a business that demanded that I work ten-to-twelve-hour days. I'm now the husband and dad I wanted to be, since I finally have more time to be with my family. Aside from having time to get the house and the yard in order, I finally have time to think about and develop a plan for the next phase of our life.

I wake up each morning grateful and refreshed. I'm inspired and feel more energized than I have in a couple of decades. The past few years were a hard lesson to learn, but they really made it clear what is and will always remain important. Real success means having time for my family. Anything I choose to do from this point forward will honor my love for them.

The sale of the business went more smoothly than I could have ever imagined. It was the perfect fit. The new owners took over something they are excited about and well prepared for, and my wife and I have been rewarded for all the hard work we've done for the last ten years. I feel joyous and inspired.

Now you're ready to write your own description. Remember, two or three paragraphs and no more than ten minutes of writing. When you're done, we'll continue with Step 7.

Step 7

Now you are ready to use the description of having your desire fulfilled to write your *sankalpa*. For this step, use your rational mind to work with what your intuition has already told you. Read over the description of your desire being fulfilled and figure out how to briefly state, in one to three sentences, exactly what you want to fulfill in the next six to eighteen months. For example, Eric read over his description and formulated this *sankalpa*: "Free at last! The business sold before the first of the year. It worked out perfectly for buyer and seller. We are all thriving." It's important to see that none of the associated words that Eric uncovered (in Step 5) appear in his *sankalpa*. Their real purpose is to provide you with what otherwise might be hidden clues about your *sankalpa*.

Drafting Your *Sankalpa*

Having completed Steps 1 through 7, you are prepared to draft your *sankalpa*. The best way to formulate your *sankalpa* is simply to ask yourself these two questions:

- What do I want to achieve or become?
- What would having it look and feel like to me?

The easiest and most efficient way to set down your *sankalpa* in writing is to imagine that you have achieved your desire; now decide on the words you would use to tell someone that you have done so.

Your *sankalpa* should be expressed in terms that can be measured—quantitatively or qualitatively. Examples of quantitative change include an increase in your income, exercising four times a week instead of one, spending more time with your family than you currently do, completing the coursework for your degree, cutting down your coffee consumption, stopping smoking, starting to save money, creating a new sculpture, or writing a play. Qualitative changes aren't as easy to measure, but if you make your goal—and your *sankalpa*—about a qualitative change in your life, you will know that you've achieved it because you will experience it. Examples of qualitative changes include experiencing a greater sense of self-worth, more confidence, more patience, more playfulness, increased creativity, increased freedom, a sense of purpose, a greater measure of faith, increased intuition, or a more viable connection to your Source or Spirit.

In putting your *sankalpa* into words, you may also want to include the emotion you would feel when you've accomplished it. An example of this approach would be a *sankalpa* such as "I'm thrilled! I found the perfect job that satisfies me in every way!" A statement like this is affirmative and clear, and it has the power to influence your thoughts, your actions, and the forces of destiny toward achieving your desires.

Your *sankalpa* has to speak to you in a voice you can relate to, so if you don't feel that you want to include an emotional component, don't. Randy, for example, didn't write about the emotion she would feel in achieving her desire. She formulated her *sankalpa* simply as "I express all of myself through self-nurturing acts," and as you've seen, it was extremely powerful and effective.

Most important, remember that while your Dharma Code describes a general principle for how you are going to approach your life, your *sankalpa* is something particular that you want to achieve in the short term.

Here is a summary of the key points to keep in mind when drafting your *sankalpa*:

1. Your *sankalpa* can focus either on the result you are seeking, the attitude that will help you achieve it, or both. You can

take either one of these approaches or combine the two. The first approach addresses a specific result, such as "I was promoted and am head of my department at Greenfield, Smith, & Smith." The second approach would address the change in attitude necessary to achieve that result. For example, you would shape your *sankalpa* around the attitude that would make it more likely for you to get the promotion you desire. You might phrase your *sankalpa* as "I am confident and self-assured. I bring the best of myself to every encounter and every opportunity at work."

2. Your *sankalpa* needs to be specific. Making your *sankalpa* specific means writing it so that the quantitative or qualitative change you want to achieve is clearly stated and that six to eighteen months from now you will be able to clearly know whether or not you have achieved it. If your *sankalpa* is about an external achievement, then your statement needs to convey that the specific thing you want has already been achieved. For instance, "The screenplay is done. I made my deadline. My producer could not be happier!"

3. Your *sankalpa* needs to be achievable in six to eighteen months. It's important, especially in the beginning, to develop confidence in your ability to achieve your goals. This is why I recommend that your *sankalpa* be something that you *know* you can achieve in the next six to eighteen months. It's okay—and I invite you—to be ambitious, to have ever-larger and more expansive intentions. But if you don't see results, especially in the beginning of your work with resolution, there's a tendency to lose faith in yourself and in the process. That's the last thing we want. Each time you fulfill your *sankalpa*, it is a victory that builds a sense of your capacity to shape and fulfill your destiny.

4. You need to believe you can achieve your *sankalpa*. It's okay to have some degree of doubt, but for your goal to manifest, at least 51 percent of you—preferably more—needs to be-

lieve that it is possible. If, for instance, you decide that your
goal is to become a managing partner in the firm where you
work, but right now you are working in the mail room, then
I would not make your *sankalpa* "I am a managing partner
in the firm of Greenfield, Smith, & Smith." It would be better to focus on an intermediate intention. Create a *sankalpa*
that moves you up in the organization, for example, becoming head of the mail room. This will help you gain confidence and help you move in the direction of your ultimate
goal. After you've accomplished head of the department, you
might then find you truly believe that one day you can become a managing partner.

5. Your *sankalpa* needs to be worded in the present tense and
   stated actively. It is essential that your *sankalpa* statement reflect that you've *achieved* your intention, not that you hope
   to achieve it someday. It should be "I got promoted and am
   head of my department at Greenfield, Smith, & Smith." I
   also suggest that you avoid the gerund form of verbs, which
   end in "ing." "I meditate every day" is much more active
   and direct than "I am meditating every day." Similarly, avoid
   a *sankalpa* like "I hope to one day heal my lower back pain."
   Instead, a better resolution would be something like "I am
   free of back pain."

6. Your *sankalpa* needs to be stated in words you would actually say. I want to emphasize the point that whichever approach you take, your *sankalpa* needs to be phrased in words
   that sound like something *you* would say. Avoid getting
   overly poetic or dramatic. Make it simple, direct, clear, be-
   lievable, and concise.

I can't say the following strongly enough: avoid a *sankalpa* that is too
lofty or otherworldly. Don't overthink it. However, if it will help you to
focus on your goal, your *sankalpa* can include the emotional experience
of accomplishing it as in the example of Eric's *sankalpa,* which began
with "Free at last!"

Below are examples of *sankalpas,* all of which have been fulfilled.

My first children's book is published and selling well!
I am a life-changing and successful clinical social worker.
My volunteer work with veterans is helping them profoundly.
My office is transformed! It is organized and allows me to be effort-
    lessly effective.
I received the grant money to do my research!
I am back to perfect health.
I enjoy my life even more because I make more time for friends,
    fun, sensuality, and adventure.
I practice meditation daily. It touches and enriches every aspect of
    my life. I feel free.
I have a partner who shares my spiritual ideals and deep love for
    life.
I am thriving! I'm down to 135 pounds, my relationship is a source
    of bliss. My career is smoking.
I am so happy and grateful for my amazing group of friends. They
    are active, healthy, inspiring, and supportive. I am living the
    time of my life with them.
Alan and I are engaged! He's moved in. I am in love and happy.

Now that you've read all of these examples, take out a blank sheet of
paper and write your *sankalpa.* Please keep in mind that the first draft of
your *sankalpa* does not have to be perfect. Once you start methodically
applying your *sankalpa,* which I outline in the coming chapters, you will
gain insights into if and how it needs to be refined.

You *Do* Shape Your Destiny

"Each thought wave influences the mind and creates therein a vibration
that affects your whole life. Each emotion affects your destiny—your
karma." This was one of my teacher Mani's favorite tantric maxims, and
it should serve as a powerful reminder to us that the vows we make,
whether constructive or destructive, whether made consciously or unconsciously, are the forces that create our world, our destiny.

Our vows, our deeply held promises, influence our body from moment to moment. They even have the power, the tantric tradition tells us,

to influence people and circumstances to come into our lives that make achieving our intentions more likely. They do, in fact, shape our fate.

What will your destiny be? It depends on you, or more accurately, on the resolutions to which you are most committed. The vows and promises you hold dear, when you are deeply committed to them, speak directly to the universe, compelling it to act on your behalf. When such conviction is linked to *dharma,* the aspiration to become the best you can be, you will be led to a life of joyous fulfillment and accomplishment. Strengthened and focused by your *sankalpa* or resolution, you will eventually learn to see how all things, all experiences—even those that are challenging or might first appear to be obstacles in the path of achieving your desire—are actually helping to guide you toward the fruits of your intention.

Throughout this section, you've worked to develop your *sankalpa.* This resolve is something your soul has led you to recognize as important. Ideally, you will treat your *sankalpa* like the precious seed it is—a seed that, when it bears fruit, will provide you with contentment and joy. In the process, you will be made stronger. You will develop faith in yourself and in your ability to shape your future. As you become more capable and powerful in the service of a higher ideal, your resolution will help you positively affect the world in which you live.

Armed with the words and feelings tied to your *sankalpa,* you are now ready to move on to Part IV, where we will begin to explore the science of how to effectively "plant" your intention and therein ensure that what your soul aspires to, can be made manifest in what are sometimes unexpected, even miraculous ways.

REFLECTIONS ON THE POSE DEDICATED TO THE SAGE VASISTHA

· · · ·

Vasisthasana

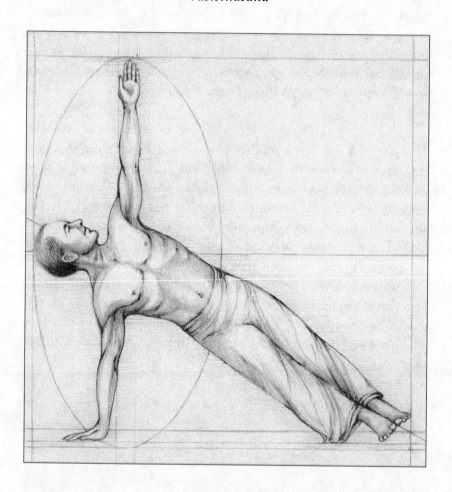

Given the great sage Vasistha's place in the Vedic tradition, it is fitting that this challenging and invigorating pose dedicated to him epitomizes grace, strength, and steadiness. The pose requires you to use your whole body—to integrate leg, back, abdominal, and arm muscles. In addition to having to strengthen these muscles, the pose also requires you to align the arms over the hand that's on the floor, and to align the front and the back of the body. Finally, you need to create a balanced lengthening from the legs through the hips and spine. However, before you can achieve any degree of alignment, the pose requires you to balance using just the hand that is on the floor and the outer edge of the back foot. Far from your body being stable, the posture deliberately destabilizes you in order to help you develop and grow past all of these challenges. Confronting all of these challenges that call upon your body to work as a whole, this is not a pose that every student will be able to do the first time he or she comes to yoga class. Even those who are strong may find it difficult to hold it steadily for any length of time. To make progress in this pose is to gain insight into the abiding principle of intention.

As with any posture that challenges you, when you first begin practicing this posture your body feels less like an integrated whole than like many separate parts, few of which seem to be working together. However, when you resolve to do your best in the posture—which means applying yourself fully to every step of getting into the pose, holding it, and letting go of self-judgment while you are in the process of practicing it—your intention becomes the organizing principle by which your various body parts gradually learn to work together. Singleness of purpose increases your capacity. By applying an intention consistently, you transform disparate efforts into unified action, chaos into order. Through informed intention you find your body—as well as yourself in the larger scheme of your life—moving purposefully, ever closer to your goals.

The pose dedicated to the sage Vasistha reinforces one of life's most vital lessons: there may be nothing as powerful in determining your future as your resolve to do so.

PART IV

. . . .

OVERCOMING
RESISTANCE

CHAPTER 11

. . . .

THE FORMULA FOR FULFILLING YOUR DESIRES

Even before she raised her hand I could tell Becky was upset. I would quickly discover why. "You know, Rod, with all due respect, this *sankalpa* thing is not working. It's been months. . . ." Her frustration gave way to anger. "I've been repeating it and repeating it, focusing on it. It's not working. I have no sense it ever will. In fact, things seem worse since I started saying it.

"I'm trying. I really am, but each time I work with my *sankalpa*, I just get pissed! It is just not working. Did I say that already? What should I do? Should I stop? Should I try a new one? Tell me, because . . ." She looked around the room at the sixty or seventy people watching her. "Well, maybe it's just me. . . ." Her voice trailed off in disappointment.

All eyes now turned to me. I had no doubt there was a solution for Becky's plight, but I needed more information before I could know what it was. "What exactly do you want, Becky?" I asked. "What is your *sankalpa*?"

Becky looked at me, hesitated, then said, "I want more patience. My *sankalpa* is 'I am patient and full of ease.' " No sooner had the words crossed her lips than she started laughing. So did everyone else in the room. Becky wanted patience, and she wanted it *now*! Not only did she not have it, but she was further away from it than ever.

Despite there being humor in Becky's plight, her frustration was real. Moreover, her inability to achieve her resolution or *sankalpa* highlights an important fact: *for every resolve, there is always at least some resistance to its fulfillment.* The amount of resistance may not be enough to keep you from achieving your goal, but unfortunately, it often is. It's one thing to have an intention; it's an entirely different thing to have that intention realized. As Becky discovered, constantly affirming your *sankalpa,* even if you've found the perfect way to phrase it, is not necessarily going to materialize it.

Acknowledging what you want and finding the right way to say it are two steps in the process of attaining it, but there are other steps in the process to make a *sankalpa* truly effective. This part and much of the rest of the book are devoted to the other steps of the process that will help you be among the 20 percent of those who wind up achieving their resolutions instead of the 80 percent who do not.

If you have completed the steps in the previous parts, you now have two keys to fulfillment. The first is your Dharma Code, a clear and defining statement of purpose to guide you in your life's journey. The second is your *sankalpa,* a specific short-term goal that is aligned with your higher purpose or Dharma Code. So you aspire to it, and through the Bliss Meditation and *sankalpa* exercise you did, you have a clear sense of what it would be like to have it. Nonetheless, it's quite possible that your desire will elude you, as Becky's eluded her, unless you apply a vital set of strategies, through which I will lead you. Becky had learned these strategies in an earlier workshop, but she chose not to use them until she recognized that merely having the intention was not enough. Doing less than the entire process, she found out, was like not really doing the process at all.

You've probably heard a great deal about the power of intention: want anything intensely enough and it will be yours; put your affirmation on your refrigerator door so you can see and reaffirm it constantly and you will fulfill what you are affirming. If these assertions are true, why is it that some things you've dearly wanted have not come to fruition?

Addressing this issue, my teacher Mani would frequently state, "Man proposes, God disposes." This quote, commonly credited to the Italian poet Ludovico Ariosto, was often the way Mani would introduce the science of manifesting intention. These four simple words, "Man proposes, God disposes," convey a timeless truth that people of all cultures are all too familiar with: no matter how hard we may try, inevitably there is a gap between wanting and having. Proposing—declaring what you want—is only the first step in what for most mortals is a two-step process. The second step depends, at least to some degree, on the universe disposing, that is, cooperating enough to fulfill your desire.

The gap between proposal and disposal can be short. If I want a breath of fresh, unpolluted air, all I need to do is walk away from my desk and go outside. Because I live in Colorado, the gap between wanting fresh air and breathing it is

> . . . .
> *No matter how hard we may try, inevitably there is a gap between wanting and having.*
> . . . .

negligible. If I were still living in Los Angeles, it would be another matter. That said, very often the gap between proposing and disposing has as much to do with internal resistance as it does with external obstacles. Fortunately, there is a methodology to help reduce both kinds of resistance to achieving what you want—in other words, to reduce the gap between what you want and what you have. Our exploration begins with something I call the Creation Equation.

The Creation Equation

The Creation Equation is a formula I devised to explain the universal principle of attainment or, in practical terms, the process of how one moves (or doesn't move) from desire toward its fulfillment. Notice I said *toward.* The moment you want something, you and the object you desire are suddenly closer, in the sense that now you have a relationship with it; however, that doesn't necessarily mean that you are close enough to have it. The methodology of fulfilling your intention or *sankalpa* is often portrayed as a deep and profound mystery. Yet this formula, the Creation Equation—which I was inspired to develop based on a teaching of Swami Rama's—makes the methodology clear and straightforward.

The formula is about the power or force behind three key elements: desire, the processes you engage to fulfill that desire, and resistance. In Sanskrit, the terms we could use are *shakti,* for the energy behind your initial impulse or desire; *vayu,* for the sum of the energy that you direct toward fulfilling that intention; and *karma,* which in this context refers to the total sum of resistance that obstructs you from attaining or fulfilling your desire, called *prapti* in Sanskrit.

The Creation Equation states that when the intensity of desire, or *shakti* (I_s), plus the intensity of the energy you direct toward achieving it, or *vayu* (I_v), is greater than the intensity of resistance, or *karma* (I_k), it equals attainment of your desire, or *prapti* (P). Thus, the formula looks something like this:

$$I_s + I_v > I_k \approx P$$

The first of these three elements is *shakti,* the force behind your initial impulse. This is the spark that lights the fire of your wish or desire. In tangible terms, let's say your desire is to complete a master's thesis. Your desire for it would be your *shakti;* attaining it would be your *prapti.* When starting toward any goal, it's crucial to clarify for yourself how much you want to achieve it, because the stronger your desire, the more likely it is that you will take the actions that will carry you to the ends you seek. A strong desire to complete your master's thesis, like any other intention, is a very good start toward achieving it, because it will provide you with more of the force necessary to overcome the challenges (internal or external) to completing it.

The second of the three elements in the Creation Equation is the energy you will invest in accomplishing your desire. This is your *vayu,* the force that your *shakti* uses to express and fulfill its intentions. *Vayu* entails all the forces you will summon physically, mentally, emotionally, materially, socially, and spiritually to help you achieve your desire. These could include any or all of the following: willpower, discipline, love, finances, networking skills, patience, forgiveness, self-acceptance, intelligence, self-study, clarity, discernment, laughter, and joy. For example, your *vayu* for finishing your thesis might require the energy to outline it, research it, and write your first draft, second draft, and even third draft. It could include the energy that it takes to eat healthfully and get enough rest, and the strength to say no to friends who might want you to hang out with them. It is also the commitment it takes to make the time to write your thesis and to accrue the finances you will live on while you write it. Finances? That's right. Money can definitely be a factor in contributing to the force of *vayu.* There are plenty of things that I am certain you would love to do (or not do), but because of a lack of financial resources—a lack of *vayu*—you find it more difficult to fulfill those intentions.

The third force in the Creation Equation is resistance: the sum of forces that limit, obstruct, or challenge you as you seek fulfillment of your desire. This limiting factor, which I'm referring to as *karma*, includes internal as well as external factors that inhibit you or that make it more difficult for you to finish your thesis. Your *karma* in the case of wanting to complete your thesis might include a lack of discipline, a noisy dorm room, an uncooperative boyfriend or girlfriend, an additional workload, the fact that you missed a week of classes relevant to your thesis or that you did not pay attention in class, and/or a lack of finances that requires you to keep working full-time. It could also include external circumstances completely beyond your control, such as the illness of a close relative or even a natural disaster.

The intensity of these three elements—desire, what you invest to accomplish your desire, and resistance—determine whether or not you will achieve your desire. Combine the total energy or intensity of *shakti* and *vayu*, and if it is greater than your resistance (*karma*), you *will* achieve your goal—every time. In the example I provided, if the intensity of the desire and the energy you invest in manifesting it are greater than your resistance, you will complete your thesis; if the resistance is greater, then you won't. Revisiting the formula, it is essential to recognize that whichever side is the greater force—either the desire-plus-energy-toward-achieving-it side or the resistance side—will determine whether or not you arrive at fulfillment of your desire.

This formula is infallible. There is no wish that has been fulfilled, nor any wish that has been denied, that does not adhere to the principle of the Creation Equation. Every time that you got what you wanted, your desire for it plus the energy you invested in achieving it were greater than the forces that resisted you having it. Each time they weren't greater, you didn't get what you wanted.

Suppose, for example, your desire is to stop smoking cigarettes. The first question to ask yourself is how much you want to quit smoking. Is it something you are doing because you think you should, because other people say you should, or is it something you are absolutely committed to making happen? Certainly the intensity behind your desire to stop smoking is key in determining whether you will be successful, but wanting it, even a lot, is not necessarily going to guarantee that you will fulfill your desire.

If you are going to successfully stop smoking, you will need to invest energy in the form of willpower, at the very least; you might also turn to exercise, diet, or perhaps a nicotine patch or hypnosis to help you achieve your desire. And you are going to have to confront the resistance to stopping. For many people, that resistance is due only in part to the physical addiction to nicotine and the other chemicals in cigarettes. For example, people often smoke to abate feelings of insecurity, nervousness, fear, and anxiety. And even when emotional and psychological factors such as these aren't contributing to resistance, some of your other habits, such as drinking alcohol, may increase your compulsion to smoke, or lower your ability to resist the urge—in which case you may have to choose to reduce the amount and frequency of your drinking.

As you can see, resistance can be internal or external; its source can be emotional, physical, financial, psychological, familial, cultural, or anything else that creates an obstacle to achieving what you want.

The key to successfully achieving your desire to stop smoking cigarettes (or to fulfill any other desire, be it material, spiritual, or emotional) is to increase the combined forces behind your impulse to achieve your goal along with the sum force you invest to achieve it and/or to reduce the forces of resistance that obstruct you from achieving it. Whatever your intention, understanding how to apply the principles behind the Creation Equation is the key to manifesting the things you desire.

The reason Becky didn't fulfill her desire to be patient was that the sum total of the force of her resistance was greater than the energy she had invested in the other parts of the equation. No individual, organization, or nation has ever achieved anything when the force of resistance was greater than the sum of the desire for a goal plus the force of what was invested to achieve it. On the other hand, consider President John Kennedy's goal for American astronauts to be the first human beings on the moon. First he instilled a passion, a desire to accomplish this specific goal, and then he inspired the country to believe that it could and should be done. The collective motivation he generated spurred needed funding to overcome the obstacles and eventually to accomplish the goal of landing on the moon (though, alas, he did not live to see the successful completion of the process he had set in motion).

The desire for world peace, however, has not been fulfilled, and the reason for that is simple: despite how attractive it may seem to those who want it and the efforts of some powerful and spiritually minded individuals who are deeply committed to achieving it, at present there is too much resistance to its happening. Until there is a significant shift at a collective level and the sum of the force of our desire for world peace and our willingness to invest significant energy to realize it becomes greater than the resistance among those who do not want it to happen, it cannot materialize.

Analyze the formula and you find that there are two basic approaches to working with the Creation Equation to make it more likely to achieve what you want. One is to increase the *shakti/vayu* side of the equation; the other is to diminish the forces of resistance on the other side. Thus, to influence the *shakti/vayu* to be greater than the *karma* side, you must (1) amplify the force behind your desire, (2) increase your willingness and the energy you invest in the processes that will move you toward fulfilling your desire, (3) diminish the force of the *karma* (resistance), or (4) do some combination of the above.

If you could implement this knowledge consistently and with sufficient power, you would maximize the chances of your desire being fulfilled. The alternative, as in Becky's case, where her desire for patience plus the energy that she invested in achieving it were no match for her resistance, is a recipe for failure. Becky's resistance was in large part due to how much her impatience had become part of her personality—and her unwillingness to let go of it. In the past it had actually served her, having become a way to avoid feelings of not being in control as well as a means to keep others at a comfortable distance. She had also used impatience coupled with rage to get people to act and respond to her, and it had indeed helped her get what she wanted.

In other words, in the past Becky had used impatience; now it was using her. The result was that her initial resistance—not all of it conscious—to being "patient and full of ease" (her *sankalpa*) was greater than the means she was using to get it. Despite her desire to be patient, Becky's goal would remain beyond her reach until she found the means to reduce her resistance and build the intensity of the means she would need to employ to achieve her desire. Not surprisingly, her way of reacting to not having what she wanted was to get impatient and angry, as she had been doing for several decades.

Becky's experience raises all the key questions that surface when we try to use the Creation Equation to manifest our intention: "How do I intensify my desire and energize the forces that will help me manifest it? What are the specific resistances that stand in the way of my fulfilling my desire? How do I reduce those resistances and make sure they don't keep me from fulfilling my intention? In short, how do I make it as likely as possible that I will achieve my desires?"

In the chapters that follow, I will answer these questions and take a closer look at each of the elements of the Creation Equation. I will also walk you through several extraordinary practices to help you apply the principles of the Creation Equation to achieve your goals.

CHAPTER 12

HOW MUCH DO YOU WANT
WHAT YOU WANT?

I've done personal consultations for more than three decades. I've met with thousands of people, all of whom sought me out because they wanted more happiness. Each has wanted to fulfill a specific desire (peace of mind, better health, a greater sense of reward in their career, making a more positive impact in the world, relieving grief, resolving struggles with a spouse, gaining more emotional balance, or learning to meditate). I've watched many achieve their dreams, often in ways far more fulfilling and meaningful than they had expected. I'd love to be able to say that every person I've advised has successfully achieved his or her dreams, hopes, and intentions, but the truth is that some have not—and in almost every instance, I've known beforehand, at the very moment that the person tells me what he or she wants, whether the person will be successful in fulfilling this intention.

I'm not a fortune-teller, but I am able to sense the intensity of people's desire for what they say they want. As we've seen, the simple rule is that when people are less than completely passionate and fully invested in seeing their dream fulfilled at the beginning of the journey toward achieving their desire, they hold less chance of being able to overcome the resistance they are sure to encounter in the process of moving toward it.

The Levels of Desire

The Vedas teach that desire has four levels of intensity. Each one is a progressively more compelling force that exerts an increasing influence on destiny. The first level of intensity is a wish (*abhilasa*), which has the least power behind it. It qualifies as desire, but in terms of sheer energy, a wish in and of itself has little of the crucial impetus necessary to move you very far toward achieving your desire. In the scheme of the energy that generates great works and meaningful accomplishments, thoughts such as "It would be nice to have . . ." or "Instead of what I have right now, I'd rather have . . ." are practically inert. This is particularly true when what you are wishing for is significantly different or distant from what you have now.

A wish can come and go in your consciousness, leaving little or no mark on creating a new and better future. I can wish to open my window, yet despite the fact that it opens very easily and is only six steps away from where I'm sitting, it still won't open until my desire for it is strong enough to get me to move out of my seat, walk the six steps, and slide it open. Even though there is hardly any resistance keeping me from opening it, wishing for it to open won't get it done.

The second level of intensity (*svatmi karana*) refers to a desire becoming important enough to influence your thoughts and actions. The Sanskrit term for this level of intensity relates to the principle that when you embrace a desire fully enough, it literally becomes a part of your *sva* or self. A common experience of this is the kind of feeling that arises when you're strongly attracted to someone or you really, really want something. At this stage of wanting the object of our desire influences the way we think, feel, and act. At this second level of intensity, you hold on to your desire consciously and with enough determination that it has become part of your nature (*svatmi*); in other words, you can't imagine yourself without the object of your desire. You, or part of you, becomes bound to the object of your desire. At this level of intensity your attention on your desire has increased to a point that is commonly referred to as *intention;* a part of you is invested in seeing your desire fulfilled. Your desire has now gathered or collected more energy and intensity for it to be fulfilled. Thus, it becomes more likely that you will achieve it.

At the second level, my desire to open the window will continue until I get up, walk to the window, and open it; but my intention may be interrupted by another intention that is stronger. Many of our desires—indeed, many of our resolutions—never get past this level. Even so, if the resistance you face is not too significant, as is the case with my desire to open my window, since there is practically nothing to keep me from doing it, then it's possible that this level of intensity may be enough to manifest your desire.

One way to understand how the strength of desire can make things happen is to think about how much more you get done when you're on a deadline, particularly when what's at stake is important to you. Looked at from the perspective of the Creation Equation, a deadline has the effect of raising the intensity of your desire to get something done. Because you want it more, you put more into overcoming the resistance, and therefore the likelihood of your achieving it is significantly increased.

The third level of desire is indomitable will and determination (*iccha bhavana*). This means becoming unwilling to fail. You won't take no for an answer. Your desire, will, and action, even your speech and thoughts, become like a laser that is focused on achieving your goal. The full force of your desire is now unyielding. No amount of discouragement keeps you from continuing to invest all of yourself and everything in your reach to attain your goal.

Elevate the intensity of your desire to this level and fewer and fewer things are able to obstruct you from achieving or fulfilling it. If I get to the window and find out that it's sealed shut, if I am determined enough I *will* find a way to get it open. At the level of indomitable will and determination, you gain access to internal resources that otherwise remain dormant but now create the momentum that allows you to manifest your intentions.

As you uncover your inner storehouse of indomitability, your sense of yourself and your capacities naturally begins to expand and evolve. You stop looking outside yourself for why you may not yet have achieved your desire. Instead you begin to generate more will, more knowledge and understanding, and you intuitively begin to act in ways that draw your desire ever closer to manifestation. You spontaneously begin to align with the boundless intelligence of *dharma*. Yet while this third level of intensity is capable of generating considerable force on the left side of the Creation Equation, in some cases—depending on the level of resistance standing between you and your desires—it still may not be enough force to achieve your desire. Going back to the example of world peace, even if several thousand people were able to generate this level of intensity toward their desire for world peace, there is still enough global resistance to it that achieving it is anything but certain.

The fourth level of intensity is mysterious and therefore the hardest to describe. Yogis call it *sankalpa siddhi,* the literal translation of which is "perfect manifestation of resolution." At this level, desire is no longer based on hope or on the point of view that you, the desirer, are separate from your desire. At the level of *sankalpa siddhi,* there is no distinction between wanting and having. It is the capacity to perform what most of us would consider miracles, when merely thinking of something is enough to manifest it. It is the state of consciousness whose effect is capable of defying what most of us consider the laws that govern the material world. It is born from the experience of complete oneness, enlightened awareness, and the highest levels of relaxation and ease.

To access it, it is necessary first to establish oneself in a unique kind of repose, a state in which one is completely whole. At this level, the lines between future, past, and present blur and your desires cross the barrier between consciousness and matter, thereby bringing your desires to fruition wholly and completely.

Manifestation—this final level of desire—is rooted in a quiet and all-encompassing conviction born from the feeling that you and the object of your desire are one. What I am describing is out of the reach of most of us, at least in the absolute sense. It is the domain of only the most exceptional of beings. India is full of stories of such beings, those who embodied this principle and could, at any time, not through trickery or sleight of hand, manifest things at will. One such story was validated by a British court, which confirmed that Bengali Baba, Swami Rama's teacher, had somehow managed to bring back to life the prince of Bhawal, who had been confirmed dead on May 8, 1909. An example from the Western tradition is the story of Jesus and the miracle of the loaves and fish, where Jesus, upon blessing five loaves of bread and two fish, was able to feed more than five thousand people.

I can't promise that you will become a master of this fourth intensity of desire. It is, however, worth looking at what the tantric tradition tells us about how you can at least begin to approach it. Why? Because to the degree that you *can* embody it, you can significantly increase your capacity to impact your future. I realize that some of you may doubt that such capacity exists for anyone. In Chapter Fourteen I will explain the principles behind it in greater depth. In the meantime, the point I want to leave you with here is that unlike the previous three levels, which can be said to incrementally increase with the application of "muscular" or willful energy, the fourth level of intensity of desire is not effortful in the common sense of the word. It is rooted in a state of complete ease and acceptance, and it is based on a unified awareness, where we are not separate or distinct from the world in which we live. Don't worry if this sounds elusive or far-fetched. In the coming chapters I will discuss in detail how each of us is capable of approaching this state and the capacities that accompany it.

What's Your Intensity of Desire?

Now would be the perfect time to ask yourself how much you want what you want. Which of the four levels of intensity do you feel toward your *sankalpa*? Is your *sankalpa* merely a wish? Is it something that you are holding a strong intention to achieve, or has it risen to the third level, where you have become an unstoppable force, truly determined to have it?

What do you do if you realize that you have less than the ideal amount of intensity to achieve your desire? In Chapter Fourteen, I'm going to lead you through an exercise that will help you gain access to desire's fourth level of intensity, manifestation, but it cannot be entirely effective unless and until you've embodied the three levels that lead up to it. Thus, before we get to the exercise, it is essential to understand

> . . . .
> *The first and most critical piece that must accompany you at every step is the decision that you cannot and will not fail in your endeavors.*
> . . . .

the first step to increase your impetus for achieving what you want. The good news is, all you have to do to take this step is to make a decision.

"Strengthen your mind and refuse to carry the burden of mental and moral weaknesses acquired in past years; burn them in the fires of your present divine resolutions and right activities. By this constructive attitude you will attain freedom," said Paramahansa Yogananda.

Whatever one aspires to achieve, whether the goal is spiritual or worldly, the first and most critical piece that must accompany you at every step is the *decision* that you cannot and will not fail in your endeavors.

Once you have taken the critical step of deciding that you fully and completely intend to achieve your desire, it is helpful to understand from where these most intense levels of desire arise. Suzanne's story sheds light on how, once you've made the decision, you can rise effortlessly through higher levels of desire and thus embolden yourself with the power to achieve your intention.

Suzanne's Story

When Suzanne came to my weeklong yoga and meditation retreat, I was surprised to hear just how utterly discouraged and lost she felt. In the past Suzanne had always seemed to radiate a sense of ease and grace. But listening to Suzanne describe her current situation, it was clear that she was stuck, lacking even a basic drive to do whatever needed to be done to improve her circumstances. For several months Suzanne had been unable to find anything redeeming about her life. There was nothing about her career, love life, or where she lived that provided her with any solace. Despite how hard she had worked and no matter how conscientious she had been in the service of her interior design clients, her business was in bad shape and she saw nothing to suggest that things would turn around. Her relationship of the past four years had ended abruptly, and she lived in a city that had been hit particularly hard by the financial crisis of 2009, a city she had wanted to move away from for some time.

What was most troubling was that she had lost all desire to do what was necessary to make her life better. In spite of the fact that she had completed the Yoga of Fulfillment course earlier in the year, she felt aimless. She managed to dismiss or discount my attempts to put things in perspective for her so that she could at least make the decision to begin moving forward in a positive direction. The good news was that she had paid to attend this weeklong retreat months earlier. This meant that for at least a week she'd spend less time brooding about her life and have time to rest, nurture herself, and clear her thoughts.

At the retreat, I made the decision not to try to help her "fix" anything. I instead intended to watch and see if and how much the practices and atmosphere of being in a retreat, away from all the things that she had so completely lost perspective on, would provide her with what she needed to move forward. The retreat was filled to capacity, so there was little time for us to speak privately. Nonetheless, I watched her and saw signs that she was gradually returning to herself. By the end of the week, the light in Suzanne's eyes had returned. A week after the retreat, I received an e-mail from her, which closed with these words: "I am again enthused, renewed, and reinspired to do the work and live my best life. The fire is back. I am impassioned and ready to make things right."

Suzanne's belief in herself and passion to pursue her dreams had returned, but not as a result of fighting with herself or trying to artificially conjure some arbitrary level of enthusiasm. Her fire was once again bright because over the course of the week Suzanne had reconnected to her source of inspiration—the light of her soul. Suzanne's transformation is a very real and practical illustration of the power of yoga and meditation to dissolve the ideas and perceptions that inhibit inspiration and our innate drive to be fully ourselves. As I described earlier, each of us is born with a ceaseless drive to thrive. The spark that fuels that drive is part of the soul's DNA. Its intensity is never diminished, but it can be overshadowed by hurt, anger, fear, grief, and our self-defeating beliefs. Yoga and meditation practice, by clearing the mind and allowing us to glimpse the part of ourselves that is an endless source of inspiration and peace, help us dissolve the accumulated stuff that dampens the soul's radiance, thereby unlocking our innate sense of passion and freedom. Thanks to seven days of yoga and meditation practice, the heavy load of despair Suzanne had been carrying had been lifted. The moment it was, she recommitted herself and made the decision to, paraphrasing Swami Rama, order her body and senses to function under the leadership of her mind.

Your soul is boundlessly impassioned and always prepared to impart to you whatever you need to thrive.

We've all probably experienced something similar. Perhaps all it took was to get away, spend time in Nature, go on a good vacation with people we love, or just be in a place we love. Any of these things can help you rediscover and reconnect to your innate drive to fulfill your aspirations.

For Suzanne, yoga and meditation provided the means to reignite her inspiration. Her experience provides an important reminder of the yoga tradition's most fundamental teaching: that you are already whole and complete. You cannot will yourself to abide in a state of fulfillment because you are already there. However, you may not be aware of it—just like the fish that doesn't know it is wet. What yoga does is to help you remove what stands in the way of your being the bright light and powerful force that you really are.

Whether or not you practice yoga, it should be comforting to know that you already have everything you need to fulfill your spiritual and worldly promise. All you need to do is purify your perception so you can recognize it. Once you do, the entire complexion of life, the world, and everything in it shifts toward sublime awareness.

That is exactly what happened for Suzanne. In retrospect, Suzanne realized that her time at the Yoga of Fulfillment course earlier that year had been less than productive because she had been so preoccupied with her old relationship that she had failed to do the critical work I'd asked her to do during and after the workshop. During the weeklong retreat, however, the rejuvenating powers of yoga and meditation enabled her to recover her love of life and self, and thus to reembark on the work she needed to do.

In the year since that retreat, Suzanne has once again come to embody a passion for living and has reclaimed her soul's desire to create her best life. This led her to reinvent herself, redefining her goals and how she relates to work and relationships. She is again making a good living as an interior designer and, although she is not in an intimate and loving relationship, she is dating again and living life with the passion, joy, and elegant manner that are uniquely Suzanne.

Inspiration is never far away, nor is it something you have to create. Your soul is boundlessly impassioned and always prepared to impart to you whatever you need to thrive. Returning to the point about *sankalpa shakti*—the importance of the decision to be a thriving and unstoppable force—it is crucial to recognize that your destiny, like Suzanne's, is to a large degree dependent on making the decision to not let your life circumstances get in the way of your goals.

We've seen the critical role of *shakti*, desire, in the Creation Equation. Now we'll look at how to make it a greater force in your life.

Intensifying the Force of Desire

My first teacher, Mani, used to say "There is only one sin—boredom." He was only half joking. His point was that if you're less than passionate about life, you are not fully alive and you've stepped out of the natural order. Boredom, anxiety, stagnation, and loss of enthusiasm are symptoms of nothing less than disconnection from your soul.

A healthy infant does not have to be encouraged to want to lift its head, to want to learn to crawl, to want to walk, then to want to run. It is compelled to do so by the sheer force of its soul's desire to be and to become. Your soul is pure, boundless creative energy or *shakti*. The closer you are to your soul, the more you abide in and embody its limitless capacities. The result is that you become more capable of accomplishing and achieving your intentions. However, as Suzanne's story illustrates, the reality is that we are not always close to our soul and therefore our fiery passion does not always burn bright. When our best intentions are not fueled by the luminous force of our passion, they can easily buckle under the weight of resistance. Resolutions are then forgotten; we respond to not getting what we want with self-doubt, apathy, boredom, and, ultimately, feelings of hopelessness.

This is one of the principal reasons that the tantric tradition places so much attention on the cultivation of dynamic energy or *shakti*. Indeed, spiritual practice, according to tantra, is centered around connecting to the limitlessly bright and fiery power that is the source of everything. In the process of building it, you strengthen the forces that propel you toward manifesting your intentions, and you empower yourself to reject those impulses that do not.

The key to intensifying your *shakti*—the initial power behind manifesting any desire as well as a passion for life—is to move closer to your authentic self. The tantric practices wholly dedicated to awakening *shakti* need to be practiced under the guidance and observation of an authoritative and knowledgeable teacher and thus cannot be properly conveyed in a book. However, I've designed the meditation practice that follows to help you easily, safely, and effectively access your soul's power or *shakti*. Practice it and you will connect to a limitless reservoir of energy and thus fuel the intensity behind your desire as well as your capacity to express it. Doing so will help expand your soul's bright light and embolden you with the force necessary to inspire and empower you, and also to sustain you through life's challenges.

Meditation to Increase *Shakti*

To do the following practice, I suggest you follow the same guidelines you did for the previous meditations: either become familiar enough with the instructions that you can lead yourself through them by memory, approximating the times; record yourself reading the instructions; listen to me leading you through the meditation on *The Four Desires* CD; or have somebody present to guide you through it.

Find a comfortable, quiet place where you can be undisturbed for the next fifteen to twenty minutes. As with any meditation practice, it is ideal if you can practice in the same place at approximately the same time as often as possible.

MEDITATION TO INCREASE *SHAKTI* PRACTICE

Position your body so that you can sit with your spine straight and your body relaxed comfortably. Sit tall, either in a comfortable and supportive chair or in a cross-legged sitting position, on a firm cushion, on the floor. Position the top of your head over the base of your spine.

Close your eyes. Become aware of your body. . . .

Relax. Feel your whole body at rest and for the next minute be aware of relaxing your entire body. Start at the top of your head and move slowly downward, relaxing and softening all tension and contraction.

(1 minute)

Become aware of the whole body and gently direct your awareness to the flow of your breath.

(30 seconds)

Watch the breath rising and falling through your nostrils. Don't force or try to shape your breath. Allow it to be completely involuntary. Just relax and observe your body breathing and the flow of air gently moving through your nostrils.

(1–2 minutes)

Become aware of the breath as two separate lines; see the breath as two separate streams effortlessly rising and falling through your nostrils.

(1 minute)

As you follow your breath for the next few minutes, continue to relax all tension in your body. Whenever you notice any roughness or even the slightest imbalance in the breath, have the intention to relax more deeply so that your breath becomes completely smooth and effortless.

(3 minutes)

As you continue to watch your breath, your mind will gradually become quieter. Just continue to watch your breath. Relax and be aware.

(1–2 minutes)

Don't force or try to make anything happen. Just relax and continue to watch your breath flow through your nostrils. In time, as your relaxation deepens and becomes more complete, this presence will become stronger and you will experience a deeper state of being.

(1 minute)

Continue to be aware of your breath; gradually begin to sense a presence in the brain.

(1 minute)

As your awareness expands, sense this presence grow. In time, feel or see it evolve into a kind of light or glow. The more you relax, the more you just allow yourself to *be* while watching your breath, the more you will experience this presence as light, unfolding.

(2 minutes)

Now begin to see, feel, or imagine a bright, golden, almond-shaped flame in the middle of the brain. Feel or envision a glow around the flame. Sense that this light or flame is a source of boundless energy and power, one that is inherently healing and inspiring.

(1 minute)

Slowly begin to allow the flame to move from your brain down the center of your spine. As it descends, notice any resistance you experience to keeping your awareness on the flame or to keeping the flame in the center of your spine. Take your time. Sense the flame moving itself down your spine; feel the inherent intelligence of the flame guiding it to descend through your spine at the perfect pace.

As it descends, feel it energizing, nurturing, and renewing the core of who you are. When it reaches the point in the spine behind your navel, see it stop and feel it become established there.

(2 minutes)

Relax and allow your awareness to cultivate the image or feeling of the flame. Sense it becoming more and more robust—a kind of living, vibrant presence in your abdomen. Sense that this flame is your source of boundless inspiration and energy. As you feel and see it, sense that you are connecting to the force that has been behind all the moments in your life where you experienced profound inspiration. This flame is your link to the times in your life where you truly excel and become an unstoppable force. For the next minute or two, sense the flame growing larger. See or feel it fill the entire abdomen, and sense its light infusing all of you with ultimate positivity and healing.

(1–2 minutes)

Now silently and slowly repeat the following words to yourself: "In me, there is a light that lights the whole world. It radiates truth: boundless will, action, and knowledge." Take your time. Be aware of how your body, mind, and soul resonate with these words. As you mentally say these words to yourself, do it with the knowledge that you are not trying to imagine something that doesn't exist; you are expressing in words the very nature of your essence or soul. Each time you say it to yourself, know that you are the embodiment of its sublime meaning.

"In me, there is a light that lights the whole world. It radiates truth: boundless will, action, and knowledge."

Each time you mentally repeat the words, pause, take them in. Feel them nurturing you, connecting you to your true nature and helping you unlock boundless capacity.

Relax. Take your time. Feel the words and be aware of them becoming more and more real to you.

(Continue for 2–5 minutes)

Finally, rest in the knowledge that you embody limitless potential and the light of boundless will, action, and knowledge.

(1 minute)

To come out of the meditation, slowly lower your chin. Before opening your eyes, rub your hands briskly together to generate heat in your palms. Then place your palms over your eyes to feel the warmth of your hands slowly energize your senses, body, and mind.

(15 seconds)

As you lower your hands and take in your surroundings, feel a quiet confidence, a renewed sense of purpose, and connected to a boundless inspirational force that is the same light that illuminates the whole world.

End of practice.

The aim of this practice is to enliven and uplift you and, as I have said, to renew your connection to your soul's inherent urge to be and to become, to seek and fulfill its fullest potential. It is a particularly useful practice during times of confusion, apathy, stress, and fear, and to renew your relationship to *dharma*.

Like any meditation practice, the more often you do it, the better. The more consistent you are and the more regularly you practice the technique, the more you will come to realize the full measure of its benefits.

CHAPTER 13

. . . .

REDUCING THE RESISTANCE THAT IS KEEPING YOU FROM HAVING WHAT YOU WANT

We've just looked at the first element of the Creation Equation, *shakti*, or desire, and how you can intensify the force of your desire to help you achieve what you want. Before examining the second element, *vayu*, the sum total of the energy you will use to fulfill your intention, we're going to turn our attention to reducing the forces behind resistance, the stuff that stands in the way of you fulfilling your goal. The more you can reduce resistance, the less energy you will need to fulfill your goal.

There are two kinds of resistance: internal and external. First, we'll examine internal resistance (mental, emotional, psychological, attitudinal). Often, your own internal resistance is enough to keep you from the fulfillment of your desires. Sarah's story is a powerful illustration of this point.

Sarah had been a longtime student of mine. Overall, Sarah had a full life. She was a creative and vibrant woman. She had a close circle of friends as well as a successful career, which, while it was not one she loved, afforded her the time to pursue what she did love—her art and travel. Although she generally felt happy, she also felt that something was missing: Sarah longed for an intimate relationship. She had not been in one for years and she was seeking my guidance with the hope of freeing herself from a long string of unfulfilling relationships.

It is no small thing to attract, let alone remain in, a nurturing intimate relationship. Few things are as wonderful as sharing your heart and entrusting your life to another. However, if, like Sarah, you grew up in a less than ideal family with an alcoholic and verbally abusive father, it's also true that few things are as challenging or terrifying.

By this point in her life, Sarah knew that if she was ever going to have the kind of relationship she wanted, she would have to overcome her pattern of either choosing a man who was too much like her father or isolating herself from men altogether. For several years, she had been seeing a therapist, as well as consulting with me once a year to update her personal yoga and meditation practice—both of which she felt were helping her move toward realizing an improved relationship with herself and possibly to her dream of a loving intimate relationship.

At our previous meeting, all her work seemed to have paid off. She seemed to have outgrown her conflicts about being in a relationship, including the worst of her fears about men. That day, Sarah had seemed practically giddy, optimistic that she was truly ready to have love in her life. For the first time, she seemed carefree. Listening to her, I found myself inspired by her lightheartedness, her progress, and her readiness. Everything seemed to be in place. Sarah appeared to be ready for the relationship she had long desired. To help her achieve her goal, I had given her a combination of deep relaxation, *sankalpa,* and meditation practices that I thought would be the final pieces to help her fulfill her dream.

It had been a year since I'd given Sarah these practices. As she walked through the door for our annual meeting, I was confident that she would tell me about being in love or, if not, that she would still be feeling very good about herself and enjoying her life. But after we greeted each other, I immediately noticed that she was not as carefree as the last time I'd seen her.

Still assuming I would hear something positive, however, I asked what had happened in the year since I had last seen her. She just sighed and said dismissively, "Oh, I've had a date or two with a couple of different people, but that's about it." We both fell silent.

I was at a loss about what to say or how to comfort her. I think she was expecting me to give her some kind of insight into what had happened. Instead, I waited. I thought it best that she share whatever insight she herself might have about her situation. When she said nothing, I posed the question directly: "Last time you said you wanted a relationship, Sarah. Today you seem to have given up. Why do *you* think you're not in a relationship?"

Without missing a beat, she said, "Oh, you know . . . the fear thing."

It was the first time she'd ever phrased her situation in that way. It was clear that she had revealed a profound truth about herself. "What fear thing?" I asked.

"Getting hurt, being rejected . . . I guess."

Her tone was nonchalant, but underneath it was sadness and a profound sense of resignation about spending the rest of her life alone. That was the moment I realized exactly why Sarah was alone. Sarah was her own biggest obstacle; she was the greatest resistance to her goal of being with someone who loved her and whom she could love.

On the one hand, Sarah wanted to be in love, to feel nurtured and cared for. She discussed it repeatedly with everyone she was close to. She spent some time every day thinking about it. That was her desire. Being in love and having intimacy was her *sankalpa*. But the more she and I spoke that day, the clearer it became that her deepest driving desire had little to do with what she thought she wanted. In fact, it was in direct opposition to it.

Remember the concept of deepest driving desire? Dean, who was diagnosed with terminal cancer, had drawn from it to lift himself out of despair and lead a life that would be an example to his son. His destiny changed almost from the moment he recognized his deepest driving desire, and he was fortunate enough to see his cancer go into remission. To repeat the scripture where the concept of deepest driving desire is found, the *Brihadaranyaka Upanishad,* "You are what your deep, driving desire is. As your desire is, so is your will. As your will is, so is your deed. As your deed is, so is your destiny."

Sarah's destiny was right there in front of us. It was the elephant in the room. If she was ever going to achieve the desire she said she wanted, she needed to admit that the elephant was standing there, taking up most of the room and making a mess on the carpet. According to this sacred teaching about deepest driving desire, Sarah was not in a relationship because her *deepest* desire, bred of fear, was to *not* be in one. She had exactly what she really wanted.

A Fork in the Wishing Road

Sarah's desire for a relationship and the amount of work she did to try to attract one were not effective because at a deeper level she was utterly committed to the opposite desire.

Sarah thought she wanted a relationship, and a part of her had a genuine wish to be in one (level one on the intensity-of-desire scale, or perhaps even level two). However, what she wanted more than anything else was something that even the best relationships cannot guarantee—absolute emotional security. Her deepest driving desire, to avoid "getting hurt, being rejected," was the desire to which she was far more committed. At some point much earlier, it had begun to be more a part of her than her aspiration for a relationship, and it could well have been a desire that had actually reached the third level of intensity. It certainly was the one that was determining her fate.

This was Sarah's "fork in the wishing road," the phrase I use to describe the place where two contrary desires meet. Given that Sarah was clinging to the contrary desire with even more intensity than to her stated goal, it was more than likely that if nothing changed, she would take the path leading her away from rather than toward the closeness and love she thought she wanted.

After some discussion, Sarah acknowledged that she did have a contrary desire. I asked her to put that contrary desire into words. I had a general sense of it, but it was critical that Sarah find a way to state it precisely. It didn't take her long: "At all costs, I want to avoid being hurt by someone I love." Given her desire to love and be loved, this may not sound rational, but rarely is resisting something we want rational—and that's just the point. That's the reason it's so important to unearth any potential desires you are holding on to that are in conflict with your *sankalpa*. Failing to unearth such contrary desires is like trying to plant a garden without first ridding the plot of all the unwanted weeds—not just what shows on the surface but the roots that descend deeply into the ground. Just as new plants in your garden can be strangled or dominated by weeds that you leave there to grow freely, it can be futile to plant an intention without first getting rid of the contrary intentions that can strangle or dominate it. With the words "At all costs, I want to avoid being hurt by someone I love," Sarah had identified what the Vedic tradition calls a *vikalpa*. You might recall that the word *kalpa*

> *Just as new plants in your garden can be strangled or dominated by weeds that you leave there to grow freely, it can be futile to plant an intention without first getting rid of the contrary intentions that can strangle or dominate it.*

means "the rule we follow above all others"; *vi* means "to separate or distinguish, to take apart, or to put asunder, division." Your *vikalpas* are the kinds of mental constructs or beliefs that split or separate you from your highest self and from the destiny that your highest self would have you fulfill. In the end, it is your *vikalpas* that make up the inner obstacles— your false ideas, deep-seated patterns, and perceptions—that lead you away from your highest destiny.

The most telling and powerful step you can take to reduce your internal resistance to achieving your desires is to identify your *vikalpas*. You may not have one that directly conflicts with your *sankalpa,* but most of us do, and even a single *vikalpa* can be a remarkably potent force, often imposing enough resistance to make it all but impossible to fulfill your dreams.

Think of a *vikalpa* as your unconscious *sankalpa,* one that moves you in any one of countless directions away from the destiny your soul is here to lead you to. It is critical to recognize that your unconscious mind is significantly more powerful than your conscious mind. This is a vital point upon which yogis, behaviorists, psychologists, and motivational speakers all seem to agree. In the battle between your conscious desire and your unconscious tendencies, the latter will win more often than not—or what probably amounts to 80 percent of the time. Indeed, the powerful and influential role of the unconscious explains why most people don't achieve their resolutions. The people who do manage to achieve them have found some way both to become aware of their unconscious patterns and how they may be sabotaging their conscious desires and to increase the intensity of their conscious desires.

Remember, your deepest driving desire determines your destiny. The pull of the unconscious and the *vikalpas* that reside there is so powerful that no matter how worthy the goal or how hopeful you might be about attaining it, they have the potential to lead you not only away from your desires, but possibly to dark, even destructive, places. The following story is a chilling reminder of just how destructive a *vikalpa* can be—and of how unearthing it can allow a new, constructive intention to find fulfillment.

Evan's Story

Evan worked in public education for ten years before becoming a middle school principal. An intelligent and disciplined professional and a devoted husband and father, he excelled at and enjoyed what he did, and he worked hard at it. Too hard—during the school year, he consistently worked sixty to seventy hours a week.

At thirty, Evan was diagnosed with hypothyroidism, an autoimmune disorder. Drugs can alleviate the symptoms, but lifestyle is definitely a factor in its onset and treatment. His medical doctor prescribed medication, rest, and less stress.

Evan took the drugs but neglected the rest of his prescription. Less than a year later, he developed vitiligo—another autoimmune-related disorder also exacerbated by stress. Again doctors told him he needed to take better care of himself. Despite the clear and ever more alarming signs that his immune system was breaking down, Evan failed to heed their advice. A year after that, he was diagnosed with psoriasis, yet another disease related to exhaustion and a weakened immune system. Most recently, before he'd even turned forty, he got his most serious diagnosis, rheumatoid arthritis.

Evan's health crisis—four diseases, all related to an exhausting, stressful, highly demanding life, and lack of rest—was no accident. Rheumatoid arthritis was the final symptom of a deeply ingrained pattern of behavior. Evan had a *sankalpa,* an intention he truly wished to fulfill: "I am healthy and happy." He had a genuine desire to get healthy, but his pattern of not taking the actions that were necessary for him to fulfill his intention of getting healthy and happy reveals something significant. Evan's destiny and actions were actually being shaped by a deep-seated and very contrary desire.

With each new diagnosis, Evan had resolved to improve his diet, exercise more, and practice techniques for relaxation or meditation. Yet for more than a decade, he didn't do any of these things. Why would someone as bright and disciplined as Evan fail to fulfill his very appropriate wish to take better care of himself? The answer is that his deepest driving desire had nothing to do with his conscious desire to get healthy.

Evan clearly had a *vikalpa,* and this unconscious, deepest driving desire was the source of his becoming sicker and sicker. Not until he did the work that I'm about to ask you to do did Evan discover what was keeping him from the health that he consciously wanted. Through this work he discovered that his unconscious deepest driving desire, his *vikalpa,* was directly in opposition to his *sankalpa.* Until Evan discovered his *vikalpa,* however, he was destined to keep making choices that took him further and further away from health. His deepest driving desire was shaping a destiny of difficulty, pain, and more and more serious disease.

> . . . .
>
> *The question is, is your deepest driving desire leading you toward the destiny you want or away from it?*
>
> . . . .

If you feel strongly enough about your desire and are committed to giving yourself your best chance of achieving it, then I strongly recommend you do the work necessary to recognize your own *vikalpas*. I cannot recommend this highly enough. Acknowledging even a single *vikalpa* can reveal exactly how and why you've run into conflict with your *sankalpa*. It may be the most important step you can take to ensure that you have the freedom and capacity to fulfill your intention. I'll let Thomas Merton, who was a Trappist monk and the author of more than seventy books, have the last word: "If you want to identify me, ask me not where I live, or what I like to eat, or how I comb my hair, but ask me what I think I am living for, in detail, and ask me what I think is keeping me from living fully for the thing I want to live for. Between these two answers you can determine the identity of any person."

Before I lead you through the exercise, consider this crucial point: all of us have a deepest driving desire. When your deepest driving desire supports your long-term happiness and well-being, it is, by definition, a *sankalpa;* when it does not, it is a *vikalpa*. The question is, is your deepest driving desire leading you toward the destiny you want or away from it? If you find yourself taking actions that are contrary to, or just less than supportive of, your goal or intention, or if you have found that it has been a struggle to fulfill your intention, then with a high degree of certainty I can say that you do have a *vikalpa*. And if you have one, the only way to reduce your internal resistance is to uncover it and acknowledge it.

Are There Any Forks in *Your* Wishing Road?

Identifying your deepest driving desire requires you to acknowledge the life you have manifested up until this moment—not the one you've wished for or are hoping to have achieved forty years from now. This means taking a critical and rigorously honest look at everything you've accomplished and *not* accomplished in your life so far. It also means taking a look at your dreams—those you've pursued and attained, those you've attempted but stopped short of fulfilling, and, most important, those you failed to act on. Recognizing how much or how little you've achieved your dreams, and how much or little effort you've directed toward fulfilling them, will point to your deepest driving desire.

The five-step exercise below will help you get a clear picture of the landscape of your subconscious. It will provide you with the possibility of redefining your life and creating a new destiny for yourself. Even if up to now you've resisted doing some of the exercises I've offered you, I strongly suggest taking the short amount of time needed to do this one. It can help save your life, as it did for Evan.

This exercise is an efficient way to arrive at the critical insight about whether you have one or more *vikalpas* and whether they are preventing you from fulfilling your conscious goals. It requires you to pause and turn your attention to what you actually have in your life right now. This invaluable examination of your life, which will take you less than thirty minutes to complete, will allow you to see whether or not your deepest driving desire is empowering you toward your intention.

The basis of the exercise is to imagine that your life is over. You are done, no longer alive; there is nothing more that you can do with what was your life. The exercise asks you to put an imaginary period on the sentence that is your life so that you can read and analyze it.

You will imagine that the space you used to occupy in the world is now empty. It is not important to know why or how you died; the essential point is that what's done is done and what's undone remains undone forever.

Next, you will look at your life as you have lived it through the eyes of a close friend, family member, or someone else you'd like to hear talk honestly about the life you've lived. This is similar to the testimonial exercise you did in Chapter Six to uncover your Dharma Code. However, this time only one person will speak about you, and instead of giving a testimonial to you as a living person, he or she will be eulogizing you. This time, as well, the person won't be talking about your life in terms of all four desires, but only the category of desire in which you want to achieve your *sankalpa*. Remember, the purpose of this exercise is to help you reduce the internal resistance that, if left unchecked, is likely to keep you from fulfilling your desire or *sankalpa*.

Before I go any further, I want to acknowledge that you are not alone if you feel some hesitancy about the exercise and having to consider your own death. Just about everyone has some resistance to imagining that he or she is no longer alive. But taking the true measure of the life you've been living is an invaluable exercise. The freedom it unleashes can help ensure that the life you *will* live from now on will be the one you truly want. Countless times over the years, students who have done this exercise have thanked me profusely for all that it revealed to them. Probably more than any other exercise in *The Four Desires*, it has changed people's lives permanently for the better.

All you need to do the exercise is a pen, a few sheets of paper, and the commitment to learn about yourself so you can live your best possible life. Let's get started.

THE *VIKALPA* EXERCISE

In a workshop, I usually give students about twenty to thirty minutes to complete this exercise.

The first step is to identify which of the four desires you, or more accurately your intuition, selected at the end of the Bliss Meditation. This is the desire that became the basis for your *sankalpa: dharma* (purpose, contribution to the world at large, accomplishments, especially in your job or career), *artha* (material possessions and means to achieve your life purpose), *kama* (pleasure), or *moksha* (awareness of Eternal Truth, true freedom, and fearlessness). You may recall Eric, who crafted the following *sankalpa:* "Free at last! The business sold before the first of the year. It worked out perfectly for buyer and seller. We are all thriving." The desire his intuition initially selected was *artha.* This was also the category of desire selected by Evan, who suffered with autoimmune-related diseases and whose *sankalpa* was to be "healthy and happy." Sarah's *sankalpa,* to be in a loving and nurturing relationship, was initially inspired by her desire for *kama.*

Once you've identified which of the four categories was the basis for your *sankalpa,* you're ready for the next step. Choose the person you want to eulogize you, based on the particular desire that you've chosen. It can be, but does not necessarily have to be, the same person who delivered your ideal testimonial in Chapter Six. The essential requirement is that the person you choose should be the one you feel can provide the most insight about you in that particular category of desire. The eulogy that he or she delivers will be full of wisdom, compassion, and caring, yet, unlike most eulogies that are delivered in front of family and friends, this one will not hold anything back that needs to be said about your accomplishments or lack of accomplishments in the particular category of desire related to your *sankalpa*. The eulogy will be a real and completely honest review of how you *have* lived, not how you would *like* to have lived. Keep in mind that this eulogy is going to be considerably different from the ideal testimonial you wrote in order to uncover your Dharma Code.

Imagine the speaker addressing the gathering of friends and family. His or her speech will be straightforward, painting a clear picture of you in the context of your *sankalpa*'s relevant desire. During the eulogy, the person may address the group, express his or her own feeling of loss, or even speak to you as though in the afterlife you could learn and benefit from these words. In addition to your actions, their eulogy takes into account your words and your thoughts about yourself and life, the beliefs and feelings that you may have kept to yourself. This person knows everything about you: what you did and what you did not do, your aspirations, disappointments, and hopes.

As you do the exercise, it's vital that, through the person doing the eulogy, you be able to admit that your sudden departure means you have left some things finished, some started but incomplete, and, despite your best intentions, others never begun. Be sure that all of these are included in the eulogy, because they are clues to whether or not you have one or more *vikalpas* and what they are.

The following is the eulogy that Evan used to uncover his *vikalpa*. Given that his *sankalpa* related to health and happiness, the speaker Evan chose—his best friend, Peter—addressed Evan's relationship to *artha*, the means necessary to achieve his desires.

No doubt, Evan was ambitious. He wanted to support his family so that they could live comfortably and that his wife would not have the pressure of working. Evan was always generous with what he had. Despite the fact that Evan had a modest income, he was able to purchase a home, but money was always tight.

Evan chose a stable career, yet failed to make much of a claim on his highest hopes for a passionate and fully awakened life. At the end of his life, Evan was just beginning to emerge as a savvy businessperson and educational consultant, but having grown up in financial chaos, Evan was still struggling financially because of the less-than-ideal role modeling his father had provided when Evan was young.

Evan's father had always told Evan that because he was smart, he could be successful financially and that this would make Evan happy and his father proud. Despite Evan's drive to make a significant place for himself in the world and earn a good living in order to prove to his father that he could, Evan wanted to get even with his father more than he wanted to succeed. Since in Evan's eyes his father equated success with material success, Evan was driven and prepared to do anything not to fully succeed in material terms and not to be fully happy.

So it was that Evan got caught up not so much in trying to take care of his and his family's needs but in avenging the very actions of the person who, when Evan was a child, never took care of Evan's needs. Thus, Evan's ambition had little authentic focus. Originally Evan's conscious intention was to use his job to help people. But unconsciously he had chosen a career that, in his father's eyes, would always be a failure. He would never be able to earn the amount of money that would impress his father, no matter how hard he worked. He tried anyway. Without realizing this, he literally tried so hard to make it something it could never be that it caused great distress to his body.

Though Evan was a really talented and conscientious educator, his inner demons made for a noisy and persistent conversation that drowned out the voices that urged him to take care of himself and to exercise better judgment. Self-hate, an intense competition with his father, and a deep resentment toward him for the wounds of a much earlier time in his life created tremendous stress for Evan and caused him to inflict great harm on his body and soul. Rather than seeking real fulfillment in his career, he used hard work to punish himself and his father even when it meant sacrificing his well-being.

From this eulogy, Evan was able to distill his *vikalpa,* which was to "gain revenge on my father by having him see me die." As disturbing as it may have been to admit, it very clearly explains the deepest driving desire that had created so much resistance to Evan's achieving his *sankalpa* to be healthy and happy and instead drove him to disease and suffering.

The good news is that once Evan identified his underlying resistance to his *sankalpa,* his life and health turned around. Once his *vikalpa* was no longer hidden in his unconscious, he became free and capable of creating a new life course and destiny. No longer bound to his *vikalpa*'s resistance to getting well, Evan began to exercise. He sought out health professionals, discovered that he had a variety of food allergies, made dietary changes, and even reduced the number of hours he worked while increasing the amount of time he spent exercising or with his wife and son. As his health and vitality returned, he decided to pursue a Ph.D. and to develop a different career in education. In the years since, he has become a highly respected innovator in education and has co-founded two award-winning schools. His new career has allowed him to do work that he loves without killing himself in the process.

Now it is time for you to write your own eulogy. As you prepare to dig into this exercise, consider the following questions. As you read through them, you might make some quick notes so that you will have them nearby when you do the actual exercise:

- What one or two outstanding memories does the speaker have of you related to this particular desire?
- To what extent did your actions reflect your wants? What did you want to do yet never manage to do? What hopes, aspirations, and intentions were never fulfilled? Why?
- What were the effects of your actions, including the ones you didn't take? Whom did it hurt?
- What price did you pay for not taking the actions that would have led toward fulfilling your desires in this category?
- How often and why did you (or did you not) fulfill the particular desire through the course of your life?
- If you failed to pursue your dream as it related to this particular category of desire (dharma, artha, kama, or moksha), what was the result or impact of not pursuing it?
- What does the speaker consider your greatest accomplishments and your greatest failures?
- Who was most helped or most hurt by your actions and in what ways?

As you intuit what the speaker would say, write as fast as you can, leaving nothing out. Write a page or two (or more if you like).

Once you finish, before moving on to the next step you may want to take a short break to give yourself a chance to process what the speaker has said. Some of the speaker's insights about you may be unsettling; they might force you to acknowledge truths that in the past you have preferred to avoid. If you feel like it, get some fresh air, relax, meditate, take a shower or a walk, or eat a snack or a light meal. Do something that will relax you enough that you are able to absorb what the exercise has thus far revealed.

This is optional; if you don't want to take a short break, don't. If you do take a break, make it a short one so that you don't lose momentum. Remember, you may be on the verge of discovering something that can truly change your life. So after no more than thirty minutes return to the exercise.

The next step is to have your eulogy in front of you, along with a pen or highlighter. As you read through the eulogy, highlight or circle the words or phrases that are the most significant in describing your life, in bringing your awareness to which of your goals in that category of desire you have accomplished and which you have not. The document you are reading holds clues, and it is your job to find them.

Here, for example, are the words and phrases that Evan highlighted in his eulogy:

failed to make much of a claim on his highest hopes for a passionate and fully awakened life . . . prove to his father that he could . . . avenging the very actions of the person who, when Evan was a child, never took care of Evan's needs . . . always be a failure . . . inner demons . . . drowned out the voices that urged him to take care of himself . . . a deep resentment . . . inflict great harm on his body and soul . . . hard work to punish himself and his father and sacrificed his well-being

As you read over your eulogy and highlight the key words and phrases, you may want to use a separate sheet of paper to make notes if you have additional insights into the motivating desires behind your actions.

Now use the highlighted words and phrases from your eulogy to identify the driving desire that has shaped your life until now. What single desire is at the root of the behavior, feelings, and beliefs described in your eulogy as the source of your present-day life circumstances? Simply put: based only upon the evidence of what you do have and do *not* have in your life today, what did you really, really want? What was your deepest driving desire? What does the evidence of your life say about the inconsistencies, if any, between what you consciously want and how, in the past, you have applied yourself?

To complete this step, you are going to be your own best friend, therapist, and spiritual mentor. Take a few minutes to study the highlighted words and phrases so you can draw conclusions about how you lived your life. The words and phrases paint a picture. Look at it and find the reason(s) that your destiny was what it was.

Once you see the pattern emerge or the thread that links all the facts, find

the words to describe it. Keep in mind that for a *vikalpa* to have significant negative consequences, it need not be as destructive as Evan's, which, if you recall,
was to "gain revenge on my father by having him see me die"; it need only be
in conflict with your conscious desires.

Karen's Story

Karen's story is an example of how even a seemingly innocuous *vikalpa*
can move you in the opposite direction of your intention.

Karen had a successful history with the processes of *The Four Desires*.
She had used the process several times to achieve her *sankalpas*. But this
time, after more than a year of trying, she had hit a wall and had been unable to fulfill her latest *sankalpa*. As mother to two young children, Karen
wanted nothing more than to give her son and daughter a good education and to raise them in a supportive, nurturing community. The problem was that she and her husband lived in a large city with very few
affordable educational opportunities for the children and at some distance from the countryside she longed for. Despite her diligence with
every step of the *Four Desires* techniques, her *sankalpa*, "My family lives
a life together that is abundant, peaceful, and simple, surrounded by a
school community that shares our core values and is connected to the
land," was little more than a dream.

Drawing upon the methods found throughout these pages, Karen
did everything she could think of to find good schools for her children
and a better community within the city, but, despite her efforts, she was
no closer to realizing her intention—until she went back to the process
and uncovered her *vikalpa*. After doing the exercise I've just described,
Karen realized that unconsciously she had been holding on to a deepest
driving desire that had been keeping her from fulfilling her goal. What
was the *vikalpa* that had been shaping Karen's life and ruling her choices
until that moment? It may not sound like much—it may not even sound
like a desire—but this simple statement was the powerful force that was
determining Karen's destiny: "Good daughters raise their children near
their grandparents." This was the "rule" she was following above all others. It is the one she was holding on to, which was keeping her and her
family from moving forward with their lives.

Once Karen realized that her subconscious commitment to doing
what she believed was necessary to please her parents—most specifically,

her mother—was preventing her from leading the kind of life she knew would serve their highest good, a sequence of events unfolded. These included an important, life-altering conversation with her mother that loosened long-held beliefs. In the end, uncovering her *vikalpa* would lead to Karen's family moving to another state, where, as she describes it, they found their "ideal life."

The following is a list of *vikalpas* from students who uncovered them by doing the eulogy exercise. As you read through them, imagine how, to the extent that any one of them was *your* deepest driving desire, it would affect your life.

"Unless I am perfect, I don't deserve to be happy."

"A good girl is quiet and powerless."

"I will never be good enough."

"The more successful I am, the less spiritual I consider myself to be."

"No one listens to me because I am not worth listening to."

"Contentment means not wanting anything."

"I am only recognized by my external titles, degrees, and deeds."

"I can never do anything right because I am my mother's daughter."

"I should stay small so that I will not outshine my sister."

"Trying to live my dreams is egotistical, delusional, and dangerous and will lead me into chaos (poverty and resentment) like my parents."

"I'm not worth knowing, so I run from life and from being known."

"I will lose my creativity if I'm healthy."

"It's easier to avoid pain than to face it."

"I am a sensible, dutiful Midwesterner, independent and alone."

"I have to do everything by myself."

"No matter what, I don't deserve it."

"Anything less than perfect isn't good enough."

"A strong, capable woman is not lovable or likable."

"I can't move forward because I am paralyzed by my past."

Learning to Let Go

Chances are good that your own *vikalpa* was established long ago. At one point in your life, it may have helped you survive or deal with challenging circumstances, but today it is no longer constructive. Holding on to something long after it is helpful is the theme of an ancient Vedic tale that illustrates how a solution from the past can later become a source of confinement and limitation.

One day a man leaves a small rural village to forage. As he walks into the woods, a powerful storm quickly descends. With each passing minute, the storm gets more intense and eventually becomes violent. With the storm raging, the man's only hope of not being blown away is to huddle behind a tree and grab hold of the trunk. The storm continues to rage all night.

The villagers awake the next morning to find that their village has been almost completely destroyed, but they are relieved that there's been no loss of life. The children begin to play among the ruins. Soon their attention turns to how they will rebuild their village. In some ways life is beginning to return to normal until someone realizes that the man is missing. As they begin their search, they hear someone in the distance yelling for help. A group of men go out to see if it's the missing villager. As they get closer, the cries for help get louder. Eventually the men stop in their tracks and start to laugh. What they see is the man who got lost in the storm the previous night still holding on to the tree. The storm long gone, he is yelling, "Help me! Help me! The tree won't let go!"

A *vikalpa* is often the destructive legacy of continuing to hold on to our "tree" long after the storms of our life have passed. In Sarah's case, the longing we all have for intimacy and love had been killed off during her childhood, when the need to protect herself from her father's unpredictability and abuse resulted in her walling herself off from any kind of closeness. But long after she left home and had ceased to need to keep potential partners at a distance, she was still holding on to that old habit. It is interesting that when Sarah finally put her *vikalpa* into words, she made it sound as though fear was holding *her,* not the other way around—like the villager who thought the tree wouldn't let him go. The same could be said for Evan's wanting to get revenge on his father, or for Karen's conviction that she had to do what she felt would satisfy her mother's expectations. Each instance is an example of what happens when we hold on to ideas long after we've outgrown their usefulness. The point is that as long as you continue to hold on to a deepest driving desire that is not supporting your best life, you are hampering your ability to fulfill your dream.

Your Dharma Code Is a Cure to Your *Vikalpa*

If, after completing the steps above, you have found that you do, in fact, have a *vikalpa,* I strongly suggest taking this opportunity to review, and possibly refine, your Dharma Code. It is important to understand that a *vikalpa,* in all likelihood, will not only keep you from achieving your *sankalpa;* there is a good chance it will also have a negative impact on the larger challenge of living your best life—in other words, fulfilling your *dharma.* However, an authentic Dharma Code is a powerful antidote to overcoming resistance so that you will be able to fulfill your life's purpose. Now that you have uncovered a clearly defined pattern of resistance, you have the perfect opportunity to make sure that your Dharma Code is as clear and effective as it needs to be.

The first step to evaluating your Dharma Code is to ask yourself, "Does my Dharma Code, in its present form, address the unconscious resistance(s) I've identified as my *vikalpa*?" Take a moment to look closely at your *vikalpa* and your Dharma Code, and consider whether or not your Dharma Code can move you beyond your resistance. One way to consider this is to ask yourself, "If I were to fully commit to my Dharma Code, would it help me break free from the negative pull of my *vikalpa*?" If you answered no, it means that your Dharma Code is less than completely authentic or that it is still too general.

Time and time again, students in my seminars are able to break through and arrive at their authentic and effective Dharma Code— which has been waiting for them all along—only after seeing it through the lens of their *vikalpa.* Thus, before going any further, if you find that your Dharma Code needs refinement, I urge you to take the step of rewording it so you can be certain that it will lead you to overcome your resistance and guide you on your path to lasting fulfillment.

EXERCISE: LISTING YOUR BAD HABITS

Before moving on to the next chapter, in which we'll work on further reducing your resistance to fulfilling your *sankalpa,* I'd like you to do this simple, but vital five-minute exercise. Please take a pen and a sheet of paper and make a list of your bad habits and all the ways you use your time or energy unproductively. In other words, list the things that you do on a regular basis that in the best of all worlds you wouldn't be doing. Don't worry about how long or short your list is; just keep writing for five minutes.

Your list doesn't need to include only your big, consequential bad habits, the very worst ways you expend time and energy. It should include any and all bad habits that you deem not to be constructive, such as watching too much late-night television, listening to hours of talk radio, spending too much time at work, gossiping, snacking on foods that deplete your energy, not exercising, or exercising too much. Other examples include checking e-mail too many times a day, drinking multiple cups of coffee per day, pornography, reading gossip magazines, or not going to sleep early enough. Simply write down all the things you do regularly that you would be better off not doing. The point of this exercise will become clear in subsequent work, but for now, just articulating your bad habits serves the purpose of making them conscious. Awareness is the beginning of change.

CHAPTER 14

. . . .

RELAX INTO GREATNESS

Soliciting the Cooperation of Your Unconscious

It was obvious that Nicole was deeply distressed. A friend of hers, a long-time student of mine, had brought her to a yoga workshop I was leading, believing that a weekend of yoga and meditation might help her.

When Nicole came to the workshop, she was at a crossroads. Suffering from severe endometriosis for most of her adult life, she had spent years trying to get pregnant. Now, after many unsuccessful attempts with fertility drugs and multiple cycles of in vitro fertilization (IVF), her doctors were saying that she had only one more chance to get pregnant. If it failed, more than likely she would never have a child.

In just a few months, Nicole would undergo her final attempt at IVF. As she faced what she knew would be her and her husband's last chance to have a child, she was dreading what lay ahead At this point, after the many disappointments of the last five years, she was more stressed than ever.

After talking with Nicole, I intuitively felt this last attempt could, in fact, be successful. However, I also sensed that her current physical and emotional state might make getting pregnant less likely. As fate would have it, I was scheduled to lead a Yoga of Fulfillment retreat just a few weeks before her scheduled procedure. I expressed my strong feeling that engaging the *Four Desires* processes could really make a difference.

Nicole came to the Yoga of Fulfillment retreat unsure how or if it would help her achieve her dream of having a child. Cutting to the chase, let me just tell you that ten months later, Nicole and her husband received the gift they had prayed and hoped for. They named her Emily.

The last time I spoke with Nicole, when Emily was a year old, I asked her which of the techniques and processes she had worked with at my workshop she believed had had the greatest impact on her getting pregnant. She immediately told me that it was Relax into Greatness, a systematic approach to complete relaxation that I will teach you in this chapter. "After you led us through the practice," she said, "I felt all the pain and burdens of the past few years dissolve. It gave me an amazing sense of freedom, and for the first time in more than five years, I truly felt that my happiness was not dependent on having a child. I would joyously and lovingly welcome a child if and when God were to bless my husband and me with one, but I finally had a sense of peace and a very clear feeling that I would be okay, whatever happened."

Nicole came away from the retreat with two pivotal skills for reducing the resistance or *karma* factor of the Creation Equation, thus increasing the likelihood of fulfilling her intention. One was a clear, positive, and unequivocal vision of achieving an intention (getting pregnant and having a child). The second was a real sense that she could be happy no matter the outcome of her efforts.

Nicole clearly wanted to have a child. The sacrifices (financial, emotional, and physical) that she and her husband had made were evidence that their desire may have been as high as the third level of intensity. However, despite the intensity of her desire, she and her husband had been unsuccessful. Once again, we are reminded that wanting something, even if it is with all your heart, is sometimes just not enough. The more you can tip the scale of the Creation Equation by not only increasing the force of your desire but reducing the resistance to it, the better your odds of achieving your goal. Nicole acknowledged that these two key learned skills I mentioned above helped her bring Emily into the world. Let's explore how.

A Psychological Shift

In *Healing Words*, a deeply thought-provoking book, Larry Dossey shares clinical proof that the mind has the capacity to heal the body. Citing the work of Brendan O'Regan, vice president of research at the Institute of Noetic Sciences, who studied the phenomenon of "miracle cures," Dossey summarizes O'Regan's conclusions in the following way:

> People undergoing radical, spontaneous, healing events "are in a different place psychologically." One of their chief characteristics is that they do not determinedly want healing; they are not desperate for a miracle to occur; they are not trying at any cost to extract a radical healing from the universe. They have a quality of acceptance and gratitude, as if things are quite all right in spite of the presence of the disease. Thus the paradox: those who do not demand healing are the ones who frequently seem to receive it.

It is no coincidence that the common psychological characteristic of those who are most likely to achieve "miracle cures" is so similar to the state of acceptance experienced at desire's fourth level of intensity. Abiding in that state of ease and freedom, you understand that happiness and joy are no longer dependent or reliant on any object or outcome to be fulfilled. Fulfillment becomes an ever-present condition.

It might seem counterintuitive that resting in an awareness of acceptance and gratitude for what *is* could be the ideal soil for planting an intention about what you *want*. But that is exactly what sages from time immemorial have told us, and what O'Regan's research confirms. One reason for this is that once you are able to access a state beyond both intellect and effort—as Nicole did through the Relax into Greatness technique, which I will share with you shortly—the reach of *sankalpa* profoundly increases, because you are now in alignment with the power of your unconscious, rather than in conflict with it.

> . . . .
>
> If a sankalpa *is going to work, it's vital to free yourself of the associations and feelings that bind you to your old patterns and beliefs.*
>
> . . . .

The tricky part about resolutions is that by their very nature, they may incite inner conflict. This is so because before you can want to achieve or become something, you must first recognize that you *don't* have what you want or that you are *not* yet what you want to become. For example, before you resolve to meet the love of your dreams and live happily ever after, make $200,000 per year, or meditate on a regular basis, first you have identified yourself as someone who *isn't* with the love of his or her dreams, *doesn't* make $200,000 per year, or *doesn't* meditate on a regular basis. Often this means that you will have a set of negative beliefs and feelings about yourself—feelings that are embedded very deeply within your psyche and your very sense of identity. When this happens, it may doom your conscious intentions to defeat.

This is what we saw with the *sankalpas* that were created by Becky, Evan, and Sarah. Becky's motivation to be more patient, for example, was rooted in her repeatedly experiencing impatience, which clearly was causing her pain. Not only was she aware that she was not a patient person, but a part of her was so identified with being impatient that her first reaction to her *sankalpa* not being fulfilled was—guess what—impatience. Sarah's *sankalpa* to be in a loving and nurturing relationship came only after feeling the pain of not having one, and Evan's resolution to be healthier and spend more time with his family came from the fact that he was increasingly ill and spending most of his life at work.

In each case, their feelings about their failure to have what they wanted were woven deep into their unconscious, providing a powerful source of internal resistance. Therein lies a critical teaching about what separates the most effective use of *sankalpa* from those that are less so. It also points to one of the main principles that distinguishes how the ancient tradition prescribed the use of *sankalpa* versus an approach that is popular today. Often you are told to simply repeat your intention as many times as you can: repeat it, repeat it, and repeat it some more until you get what you want. If you don't get it, it's because you failed to repeat it enough times. This approach failed to help Becky achieve her desire, just as it has failed countless others. The fact is that, according to the ancient tradition, your *sankalpa* becomes truly powerful only when you let go of all negative associations related to your *sankalpa,* including any doubts you may have about it. Until then, it doesn't matter how many times you repeat it.

Here's the point: if a *sankalpa* is going to work, it's vital to free yourself of the associations and feelings that bind you to your old patterns and beliefs, the very things that have played such a significant part in determining your fate until now.

In other words, without a repository of new, affirmative associations, feelings, and images related to fulfilling your *sankalpa*, you may find it all but impossible to fulfill it. Without this step, your *sankalpa* is limited to being a *conscious* intention, one that your unconscious may still be far from helping you achieve.

One reason I asked you earlier to write about what fulfillment of your *sankalpa* would look and feel like is because of the crucial role the unconscious plays. A *sankalpa,* the words that describe what you want to achieve, is the language of your conscious mind. You and I use words to convey information to each other, but the information that words are capable of conveying barely penetrates beyond the conscious mind. On the other hand, the language of the unconscious is *feelings* and *images,* not words. To make change happen, you have to do the work to clear or reset your unconscious. Psychotherapists know this, which is why they often try to decipher their patients' unconscious patterns and unresolved issues by exploring the images and feelings that unfold in their patients' dreams. And by writing about what having your *sankalpa* would look like (image) and feel like (feeling), you, too, are gaining access to the workings of your unconscious.

The key to soliciting the unconscious and learning to align it with our conscious intentions is knowing how to bridge conscious intentions to your unconscious mind. Without this link, repeating a conscious intention such as "I am patient and full of ease" may serve only to stoke the fire of impatience. This is exactly what happened to Becky. It's no accident that for several months Becky was unsuccessful in achieving her *sankalpa.* Later, I learned why she hadn't transformed her impatience; she had been trying to take a shortcut in the process. Becky had the right *sankalpa* but was repeating it without the right preparation. Being an impatient person, she had skipped the potentially life-changing technique of Relax into Greatness, the technique that Nicole felt contributed so much to her becoming pregnant and which I will lead you through below.

Relax into Greatness

The longer we live, the more experiences we accumulate. Some are pleasant, some are relatively neutral, and others are unpleasantly stressful. Left unresolved, all negative stressful experiences remain stored indefinitely in our unconscious. The various feelings, memories, and sensations related to unpleasant stress have a negative impact on your mind and how it relates to the world—and also affect your health and physical well-being. Multiple studies have proven the causal connection between chronic stress and high blood pressure, insomnia, a weakened immune system, diabetes, depression, and Alzheimer's disease.

Moreover, the latest research shows that stress can rewire the brain in ways that perpetuate stress. Specifically, scientists have found that when we undergo chronic stress, "regions of the brain associated with executive decision-making and goal-directed behaviors" become atrophied, "while, conversely, sectors of the brain linked to habit formation" grow as a result of stress. In other words, the cumulative effects of stress make it less likely that you will be able to escape the habits that prevent you from acting in your own best interests, and less likely that you will have the cognitive awareness necessary to achieve your goals.

The good news is that your brain is elastic. When it experiences enough of an interruption between stress cycles, brain function returns to a state that supports total well-being. This is where relaxation comes in. An ever-expanding body of research is showing the vital role of relaxation, which at one time was thought of as being little more than a luxurious indulgence or a mystical pursuit.

Thousands of years ago, the tantric tradition had already recognized the significance of relaxation. Ancient texts such as the *Vasishta Samhita* and *Sushruta Samhita* outline a detailed approach to systematic relaxation as an essential practice for maintaining health and vitality. This ancient practice was called *yoga nidra*. The word *nidra* means "sleep." *Yoga nidra* can be best summed up as "yogic sleep," which effectively means the deepest state of rest possible (complete effortlessness), combined with awareness.

The sages first developed *yoga nidra* through a profound understanding of the subtle systems that link the physical body, the mind, the energy body, and the layers of the unconscious to the soul. *Yoga nidra* was their ingenious methodology for healing and transforming each of the layers that the soul inhabits. In other words, *yoga nidra* is a complete and holistic approach to restoring and renewing the body, the mind, and the most subtle realms of being. It is also a highly accessible technique for anyone of any age.

I was introduced to *yoga nidra* more than thirty years ago by my first teacher, Mani. I later studied and practiced additional approaches to it with Panditji. From their teachings, I evolved the practice of *yoga nidra* into what I call Relax into Greatness. Almost every day I receive e-mails from those whose lives it has touched, people from every walk of life who share with me how much it has impacted their life as well as how powerful and effective and how easy and pleasurable it is to do.

> . . . .
> *The cumulative effects of stress make it less likely that you will be able to escape the habits that prevent you from acting in your own best interests.*
> . . . .

The miracle of Relax into Greatness is that the practice doesn't require you to *do* anything, which is why it can be used by anyone at any level of fitness, including those who are infirm. For thirty minutes or so, you simply rest on your back while you are guided through steps that lead to ever-deeper states of relaxation. The methods that lead you there include body and breath awareness, visualizations, and ultimately, during the final stages, learning to abide in your soul and experience awareness of your connection to the Infinite.

When I first began teaching Relax into Greatness, few Westerners had heard of, let alone experienced, the practice of *yoga nidra*. Now, two decades later, it is being increasingly embraced and recognized as one of the most powerful yogic tools both for healing and for realizing your fullest potential.

Recently, *yoga nidra* has been studied in clinical settings. In practically every case, initial findings suggest that it is a remarkably effective method to treat various afflictions ranging from sleep disorders to chronic pain, chemical dependency, anxiety, multiple sclerosis, and even low self-esteem. Some of the most promising results have come from research conducted at Walter Reed Army Medical Center and the Miami Veterans Affairs Medical Center for veterans suffering from post-traumatic stress disorder. Thanks to the success of early clinical trials, the U.S. government is currently considering funding multimillion-dollar follow-up studies on *yoga nidra*'s effect on PTSD. Additional studies are also underway at Brooke Army Medical Center as well as VA medical centers in Washington, D.C., and Chicago. The results of the studies on PTSD are particularly interesting, as they appear to validate what the teachings of tantra have asserted for centuries: *yoga nidra* is more than a way to transform the body, it is a profound modality to transform the unconscious.

Neuroscientists say that *yoga nidra* helps us access theta waves, the brain rhythm that signals the deepest rest. But unlike the theta state, which normally occurs for about fifteen to twenty intermittent minutes during eight hours of deep sleep, *yoga nidra* provides a systematic approach to access it directly. This is why the ancient teachings suggest that one hour of *yoga nidra* is the equivalent of two to three hours of normal sleep. Another major difference between sleep and *yoga nidra* is that while you are resting in the latter, you simultaneously experience complete effortlessness while being fully conscious. This means that Relax into Greatness is a complete practice unto itself, one that offers an astounding array of physical and mental benefits. Among them is that it is a wonderful preparation for deep and restful sleep. I've even heard from many people with a history of sleep issues that Relax into Greatness is a profoundly effective means to fall asleep more easily and to experience a more restorative sleep.

Through the depth of the relaxation it provides, Relax into Greatness makes it possible to unwind your unconscious; thus it is the perfect practice to combine with *sankalpa,* or resolution. Remember, a *sankalpa* is a precious seed. As with any seed, how you plant it can make all the difference in its yield. One of the most vital considerations is the quality of the soil in which you plant it. No matter how perfect the seed of your intention is, if the soil of your unconscious is packed with layers of tension and negative associations related to your *sankalpa,* then no matter how many times you water the seed by repeating your *sankalpa,* the soil will remain too hard to allow the seed to grow and bear fruit.

Too often, the accumulation of past hurts, attachments, aversions, addictions, and self-doubts subverts our goal of achieving at least some of our desires. It is important to recognize that at some point after committing to changing the course of your life, you will need to unchain yourself from your past. Your unconscious will often resist. It will attempt to maintain the status quo and therefore interfere to keep you from creating the new and different future you seek. It may tell you that you can't do it, find reasons for you to stop trying, create distractions, or generate various kinds of self-sabotaging behavior. This is why it is necessary to clear your unconscious and enlist it to work on your behalf in supporting your *sankalpa*. Relax into Greatness is the ideal method to accomplish this. When you become established in complete effortlessness and ease, where past and future burdens are dissolved, your unconscious becomes more open and available to respond to your conscious desires.

If I had to identify the single reason that as many as four out of five of us fail to fulfill our resolutions, I would point to the lack of alignment between the positive goals of our conscious minds and the negative patterns of our unconscious. The technique I'm about to teach you will, along with reducing conscious stress, renew you physically and emotionally, and help you empty the unconscious of stress so that it can release its negative patterns and conscious and unconscious wishes can fall into alignment.

Here are some hints about how to practice Relax into Greatness:

- Practice it in a quiet place where you will not be distracted or disturbed.
- If possible, draw the curtains or cover your eyes with something soft (be sure it is lightweight) so that you will experience as little sensory stimulation as possible.
- Wear loose, comfortable clothing. You may want to cover yourself with a light blanket. Be sure that you will be warm throughout the practice.
- Lie on a comfortable (not too hard, not too soft) surface.
- Consider using a folded blanket under your knees to support your lower back or a cervical/neck pillow to support your head and neck.
- Do not move once you begin to practice, so be as comfortable as possible when you begin.
- In order to derive the maximum benefit from the practice of Relax into Greatness, have the intention to remain awake throughout the process.
- If you do fall asleep while practicing it, don't worry. This is a natural occurrence, especially when you first start practicing, and particularly if you are fatigued (as most of us are at one time or another). Preventing yourself from falling asleep may be something that you will need to train yourself to do. The more often you do the practice, the sooner you will master the state of relaxed wakefulness.
- On those occasions when you do find yourself becoming sleepy, or if you are using it to help you fall asleep, make a conscious decision to stop practicing Relax into Greatness *be-*

fore you drift off. Turn off the recording, stop going through
the steps, and simply tell yourself that you are now going to
go to sleep.

- If during the practice you find yourself feeling agitated or too
restless to practice (this is a very rare occurrence), stop practicing. Make a point of practicing the next day or, if that is
not possible, as soon as you can.
- Wait at least two to three hours after eating before you do the
practice.
- Remember: don't *try* to accomplish or to *do* anything. The
state of Relax into Greatness is defined by complete effortlessness coupled with awareness. Cultivate a feeling of non-doing
even while following the directions.

You are now ready to do the Relax into Greatness practice. I am assuming that by now you have the precise
words of your *sankalpa* and you've had
some time to live with it. You may have already refined it once or twice. But don't
worry; you don't have to have the perfect
sankalpa to apply it during Relax into
Greatness. The practice of systematic deep
relaxation will itself, as it is repeated over
time, awaken your intuitive abilities and
provide you with the sensitivity and clarity
to find the precise words that convey your
heart's resolve or *sankalpa*. Thus, whenever

> . . . .
>
> *When you become established
> in complete effortlessness and
> ease, where past and future
> burdens are dissolved, your
> unconscious becomes more
> open and available to respond
> to your conscious desires.*
>
> . . . .

you use your *sankalpa* with Relax into Greatness, make note of how your
sankalpa feels. If it feels less than authentic and inspiring or if you find
your *sankalpa* hard to remember, make time afterward to either shorten
it or adjust the language so that it feels just right.

I recommend you do this practice by listening to a recording of it so
that you can be completely effortless and not have to think or consult instructions during the process. As with the other practices, either purchase
The Four Desires practice CD from www.rodstryker.com or create your
own recording of it based on the script that follows. If you record it for
yourself, be sure to speak clearly and slowly and emphasize a feeling of
complete effortlessness.

THE RELAX INTO GREATNESS PRACTICE

To begin the practice, lie down on a bed, a carpet, or a well-padded yoga mat and settle on your back. Be sure that whatever you're resting on is soft, yet supportive enough so that for the next half hour or so you can be completely comfortable and can lie still without having to move or adjust your position. You can place a rolled blanket under your knees for additional lower back support, and consider using a cervical pillow to support your neck.

When you're lying down, position your head so that your neck and upper spine are completely free of tension. Rest your arms by your side with your palms turned faceup and nothing touching your fingertips. Slightly rotate your arms toward your body so that your thumbs are just a bit higher than your little fingers. Feel your whole body opening to the earth below you.

(Pause)

As you listen, just allow the directions to wash over you. The more effortless you can be, the better. There's nothing to reach for, nothing to accomplish. Remember, Relax into Greatness is not so much something you *do* as something you *feel*. It is yogic sleep, which means the deepest state of rest with only a trace of awareness. Simply relax and be aware . . . it is all about being effortless.

Close your eyes. Let your body open and settle deeply and completely. Relax. Allow your upper and lower teeth to part slightly.

Begin by taking a few slow, comfortable breaths. Each time you exhale, feel the body relax even more deeply. Continue to breathe in smoothly, and as you exhale, release all stress and tension. Remember not to *try*. Be effortless. Repeat this for another few moments. Just relax and be aware of your body breathing.

Feel yourself dropping into a state of complete effortlessness. . . .

(1 minute)

Allow your breath to become involuntary. Sense your body now at ease, your mind open and at peace. Feel your body opening to the earth, feel your body soften. Feel facial muscles relax, jaw, tongue, and lips all relax. Even your eyes settle into their sockets. Sense that you are being nurtured by your surroundings. Feel a growing sense of peace.

(Long pause)

Before you repeat your *sankalpa* or resolution, take this moment to feel a sense of gratitude. Be grateful by completely embracing and accepting the gift of life. Feel grateful for everything that has led you to this moment, grateful for all actions, events, and decisions. You accept with gratitude everything that has led you to this moment.

(Pause)

Now it's time to work with your *sankalpa*. Begin by acknowledging that your resolve—what you aspire to achieve or to become—is in the service of something bigger than you or your life. Acknowledge that you are part of and an expression of a timeless being, the One Reality that pervades everything. . . .

In the context of this One Reality of which you are a part, begin to recall your *sankalpa*. Even before you mentally say your *sankalpa*, create the visual and emotional sense of it as a reality. Feel all the feelings related to its coming to full fruition. Imagine you have exactly what you want. Feel it. . . .

As image and feeling merge, mentally repeat your *sankalpa* three times. State it clearly and with the conviction that it has been fulfilled. As you repeat it, also feel a real joy or satisfaction, even a sense of wonder, for having achieved your resolution. Mentally and with conviction, repeat your *sankalpa* three more times.

(1 minute)

When you have finished repeating it three times, give thanks. Feel grateful that you have achieved your desire.

(20 seconds)

Now you're ready for the next stage of Relax into Greatness—a scan of points throughout the body. As I guide you to these points, do not try to concentrate on them. Simply be aware of the specific area I'm directing you to; be mindful of it while you continue cultivating complete effortlessness.

Please bring your attention to the point between your eyebrows . . . to your throat . . . be effortless . . . to your right shoulder . . . right elbow . . . be effortless . . . right wrist . . . tip of your thumb . . . right index finger . . . effortless . . . middle finger . . . ring finger . . . little finger . . . move into your right wrist . . . effortless . . . elbow . . . shoulder . . . and throat. . . .

Please go to your left shoulder . . . effortless . . . left elbow . . . effortless. . . .

Wrist . . . thumb . . . index finger . . . middle finger . . . relax the left ring finger . . . little finger . . . left wrist . . . elbow . . . left shoulder . . . and then the throat . . . all effortless. . . .

Drop down to the center of the breastbone, relax . . . right chest, relax . . . center of the chest, relax . . . left chest, relax . . . center of the chest, relax . . . your throat, relax . . . point between your eyebrows, relax . . . relax your whole body . . . relax your whole body. . . .

(1 minute)

Now you're going to cultivate different sensations.

Imagine that the body is very heavy. Feel as though your whole body is sinking into the earth. Every part of the body, arms, legs, torso, and head, is being drawn toward the center of the earth. Even the eyes and eyelids are heavy. Feel the whole body heavy. Keep feeling that the whole body is incredibly heavy. Intensify the feeling of heaviness.

(20 seconds)

Now feel the whole body is weightless. Feel the head weightless. The right and left palms are weightless. The whole body is weightless. The body is so light that you are now aware that there is space between your body and the surface on which you are lying. Create this space and feel weightlessness.

(20 seconds)

Now the whole body experiences cold. Feel cold overtaking your whole body, as though frigid winds are penetrating your flesh. Even the core temperature of the body is dropping. You're consumed by freezing cold. Cultivate an intense feeling of cold.

(20 seconds)

Now imagine heat. Imagine the body surrounded by an overwhelming heat, as if you are lying in the bright sun at midday, next to a roaring fire. Your body is overwhelmed by intense heat; you experience a profound sense of heat.

(20 seconds)

Bring your attention to the space in front of your forehead . . . about six inches in front of your forehead. Imagine this space as the screen of the mind. It is a screen of consciousness, where all dimensions of the mind can be seen and known. On that screen, visualize the color blue . . . see blue . . . visualize white . . . see the screen of the mind white . . . see the color gold fill the screen of the mind . . . gold, see gold . . . see the screen of the mind emerald green . . . see the screen of the mind violet . . . now see the screen of the mind rose . . . screen of the mind rose . . . screen of the mind violet . . . see the screen of the mind green . . . now see gold . . . see white, see white . . . now blue . . . screen of the mind black . . . see black on the screen of the mind. Imagine that the screen of the mind is empty because you are empty of all intention and effort. Your senses have withdrawn. You are effortless. As you relax and observe that space, witness any shapes or colors that appear on the black, empty screen of the mind.

(1–2 minutes)

Allow thoughts and impressions to spontaneously unfold on the screen. There is nothing to do, nothing to look for. Be effortless and just observe. The more you relax, the more likely it is that you will begin to see images unfold on the screen of the mind. Don't try. Just relax. There is nothing to look for, nothing to accomplish. The more you let go, the more your unconscious will unfold and manifest as memories and perceptions in the form of various images on the screen. Don't try, just watch.

(2 minutes)

Please bring your attention to your breath, and see the breath moving through the right and left nostrils like two separate flows . . . totally effortless, just watching your breath . . . see the breath rise and fall through the nostrils . . . relax and be aware of the breath. . . .

(1 minute)

Remaining completely relaxed, begin to visualize alternate-nostril breathing without forcing . . . see the breath rise through the left nostril, fall through the right . . . on the next inhale it rises through the right, on the exhale it falls through the left. . . .

Continue to sense the breath moving alternately through the nostrils. . . .

(30 seconds)

Please add one more step: while you breathe alternately through the nostrils, please count backward. Begin at the number fifty-four. As you inhale, you can say to yourself, "In the left fifty-four, out the right fifty-four" . . . next breath, "In the right fifty-three, out the left fifty-three" . . . in the left fifty-two, out the right fifty-two . . . in the right fifty-one, out the left fifty-one . . . completely relax, continue counting backward while visualizing alternate-nostril breathing. . . .

Continue for about five minutes. If you get to zero before I tell you that the five minutes is up, start over with fifty-four. If you lose track while counting, begin again at fifty-four. Effortlessness, counting, and alternate-nostril breathing . . .

(3 minutes)

Return to your breath . . . it doesn't matter what number you are on or if you finished . . . stop counting backward.

Move your attention to the black screen of the mind in front of the forehead . . . just observe, without getting involved, whatever comes onto that screen . . . if nothing comes, that's fine, but you will probably find that as you relax more completely, you will begin to experience different shapes and colors. This is just the unconscious manifesting. Watch, relax, and let it unfold.

(2–3 minutes)

Now see a golden egg . . . in front of your forehead, see a golden egg . . . then feel a ray of gold light from the golden egg move in through the point between your eyebrows, and feel it flood the brain . . . the whole body floods with golden light . . . the body now becomes so full of golden light that it creates an aura of gold around the body.

(1–2 minutes)

Finally, become aware of the "witness." Be aware of the part of you that has been observing the whole process of Relax into Greatness. You are now aware of being, only being and awareness. Only it is not you or your individual being, it is universal Being, unconfined, unbounded, timeless. There is no more "I," no individual self . . . there is only the Infinite, the One.

(1–2 minutes)

Become aware of the breath . . . be aware of the body breathing. You are now going to repeat your resolve, your *sankalpa*. Begin by reestablishing a feeling of gratitude . . . rest in the appreciation that everything is just as it should be . . . be in total acceptance and gratitude.

Now recollect that your *sankalpa* is in the service of something sacred. Acknowledge that you are part of and an expression of a timeless being, the one reality that pervades everything and that your *sankalpa* is part of it.

Visualize and feel the fulfillment of your *sankalpa*. Imagine you have exactly what you want. Now, mentally repeat your *sankalpa* three times. Feel the certainty that your *sankalpa* is fulfilled. As you repeat it, be aware of real joy or satisfaction for having achieved your resolution.

(1–2 minutes)

When you have repeated your *sankalpa* three times, give thanks. Feel thankful for having achieved your desire.

(20 seconds)

Slowly come back to your breath . . . come back to the body . . . begin to gradually become conscious of the sounds around you . . . take your time . . . start to move your body and then roll over to your right side to adjust . . . when you are ready, sit up . . . the practice is complete.

Some Frequently Asked Questions about Relax into Greatness:

How often should I practice? The more often, the better; a minimum of two or three times per week is ideal.

What if I fall asleep every time I practice? You probably need the rest. It may take a few weeks or as long as six months or more, but consistent practice will gradually provide your body with the rest it needs. Within a few months, you'll most likely find that you're able to stay awake consistently; the more often you practice Relax into Greatness, the less you will be prone to falling asleep. It will also help if you do not do the practice after vigorous exercise or at bedtime, and remember to wait at least two to three hours after consuming caffeine or your last meal.

When is the best time to practice Relax into Greatness? Whenever you can. In time you will find your favorite time to practice. Mine is in the afternoon, before dinner.

Parts of Relax into Greatness, the colors and the body parts, seem to go by so fast that it is hard to keep up. Am I doing something incorrectly? I go fairly quickly to make it more difficult for you to work too hard and to keep your mind from wandering. We usually hold on to an image or idea somewhere in the neighborhood of one to three seconds; after that your mind has to work to stay focused. Just listen, be aware, and relax.

Is it normal for people to get anxious or restless during the practice? It's extremely rare, but anyone can experience restlessness at some point. Usually by the next day you will be more than ready to be led through the practice again.

The Hidden Resistance Exercise

Before moving on, it's worth taking a last look at what internal resistance may be in the way of you achieving your *sankalpa*. You've already done the work of identifying your primary internal resistance to your intention, but it's important to recognize that you may have more than one *vikalpa*. Your additional *vikalpas* may not be as deep-seated or as powerful as the one that you have identified; on the other hand, they may be even more powerful since any additional *vikalpas* may be buried more deeply in your unconscious. In either case, all *vikalpas* contribute to the overall intensity of your internal resistance. Therefore, here is a quick exercise to help you identify any additional resistance or subconscious patterns that, if left unacknowledged, can get in the way of fulfilling your *sankalpa*. These minor *vikalpas* are often resolved by the regular practice of Relax into Greatness, but seeing and acknowledging them is a vital step to overcoming them.

Please take out a pen or pencil and a sheet of paper. For the next five minutes, I'd like you to write your *sankalpa* over and over and over again. Use the exact same words each time. Notice how you feel as you write the words. As long as you can believe or feel positive about what you're writing, continue to do so.

The moment you hear or sense any objection, disbelief, or resistance to your *sankalpa,* write down that opposing thought or resistance instead of your *sankalpa*. Write it down as clearly and specifically as possible, but keep it short—write down just the initial thought or feeling. Be brief. The point of the exercise is to give voice to your subconscious resistance to your *sankalpa*.

Don't analyze your objections; just write down whatever comes up. You may wind up writing the same opposing phrase or sentence more than once. That's fine. If you perceive any resistance, just write it down. If, as you're writing, it feels like you're writing more objections than you are your *sankalpa,* don't worry about that, either. This is the time to get *all* your objections, resistances, and negative ideas out into the open.

If, at any point during the exercise, your subconscious starts to rattle off thoughts like "No way," "I don't believe it," "I can't do it," "There's no chance," "It'll never happen," "I don't deserve it," or "Who do you think you are?" write all of that dialogue or as much of it as you can. Then, for the remainder of the five minutes, write your *sankalpa* again and keep writing it unless you hear or feel more objections to it, in which case write those.

When the five minutes is up, you've completed the exercise. That should be plenty of time to get the majority of your supplementary *vikalpas* out into the open.

Don't worry or get overly concerned about what you might have discovered. The intent of the exercise is primarily to have you acknowledge your resistance, conscious and unconscious, and to once again remind you of the need to energize your *sankalpa* and to intensify the forces that you are directing to achieve it so that they are greater than the intensity of resistance.

In the next chapter we move further into the process of increasing the intensity of the force (*vayu*) that leads to fulfillment of your resolve or *sankalpa*.

CHAPTER 15

BUILDING MOMENTUM TO ACHIEVE YOUR *SANKALPA*

The Departure Point

Paramahansa Yogananda observed that "success is hastened or delayed by one's habits." This is not just an abstract philosophical observation; it is the basis for two very practical methods I developed to help you increase your capacity to achieve any *sankalpa*. The first of these techniques, which I call the Departure Point, is a simple and extremely powerful method to generate more momentum toward fulfilling your *sankalpa*. The second technique, Seeding the Gap, which I will teach you to apply in conjunction with the Departure Point, allows you to plant your intention in the most effective way to fulfill your desires.

When I first started teaching yoga, it was hard not to notice that students tend to practice in the same spot every time they come to class. The first time they enter the classroom, they carefully consider their options before putting their mats down. They take in the room, measuring their surroundings to find the best place to practice. The next time, they usually drop their mats in the exact same spot. Years later, most students are still practicing in the very same spot they took the first time they came to class.

Habits start innocently enough; rarely does it occur to us that even a harmless habit may be affecting our future. Where you place your yoga mat may seem inconsequential, but the fact that you are so faithful to that or to any other habit conveys an important lesson: *your past exerts it-*

self on your present. If you don't consciously choose the direction of your life, your past will choose it for you.

In other words, if you want to change your life, you need to make a conscious choice to change some of your habits, or else the momentum behind those habits will, more than likely, propel you to the same life that you have been leading up to now.

Yogis have long emphasized the importance of avoiding unconscious action, of not doing things simply because they are familiar or habituated. Indeed, if we are not hypervigilant, we remain creatures of habit. Do something more than once and if it's comfortable or satisfies a need, there's a good chance you'll do it again . . . and again . . . and again. In no time at all it has become a habit, one that it will take effort to break.

Even trivial habits—such as watching television after work or consistently being late to appointments—are often rooted in something deeper and can hinder your progress toward making lasting change. Frequently we do these things for reasons other than our interest in the fate of the characters on our favorite TV show or our casual relationship to time. Being consistently late, for example, can be symptomatic of a fear of accountability, a way to reinforce your self-importance, or a reflection of your belief that you're not important enough for anyone to care that you're late. Thus, a simple habit may be your way of responding to deeper impulses. But as long as you continue to repeat a habit, or any nonconstructive pattern, it's almost impossible to know what is behind it or how it may be affecting your life. For example, often only after an alcoholic has stopped drinking can he or she discover the causes that gave rise to the drinking. The momentum of habitual action doesn't allow for the pause that would otherwise provide clarity, and it perpetuates the likelihood that you will continue to have what you have had (or not had) in the past. Therefore, even seemingly innocuous habits are worth reexamining.

> . . . .
>
> *If you don't consciously choose the direction of your life, your past will choose it for you.*
>
> . . . .

The most direct route I've found for enabling people to effect real change in their lives is to break a habit—not necessarily even a habit that seems in any way related to the more basic change they want to make, but simply any habit that they recognize as being unhealthy or counterproductive.

I realize that giving up a habit is not easy, but the fact is that stopping even a simple habit can provide you with the opportunity to create or attract a different future. That is reason enough to try it, isn't it? The fact that you may feel some resistance to stopping it is also a signal that there is untold power in sacrificing your habit for the sake of something you really, really want.

The Departure Point is a juncture where you break the momentum of your old trajectory by interrupting a habit pattern, and thus trigger a new trajectory toward your goal. The Departure Point technique is based on the principle that by giving something up, you create an opportunity for the universe to fill the resulting gap with something new, and specifically something you desire—your *sankalpa*. By creating space, you allow the abundance of the universe to flow toward you more easily. By stepping away from the momentum of your past, you spark the possibility of seeing and acting differently, thereby increasing the likelihood of creating a different future. It may not sound significant, but letting go of a habit and placing your intention into the space vacated by that habit can change your life forever.

Patty's Story

Patty came to my Yoga of Fulfillment workshop with no specific goal in mind. At the point in the course where her story begins, she had done all the work I've already walked you through. The desire that came out of her Bliss Meditation was *kama,* the desire for pleasure. However, to her surprise, when she did the exercise to discover the associated words, *anxiety, fear, worry,* and *frustration* came up. Looking at these words, which all describe feelings of discomfort, she realized that she tended to push away or deny many of her feelings. Processing this, she recognized that she needed to become more conscious of her feelings if she was going to be led to fulfill her desire for more *kama* or pleasure.

This led her to the following *sankalpa:* "Always mindful of all my feelings and thoughts, the peace within me bears real fruit." Frankly, I wasn't sure that she had created the ideal version of a short-term goal or *sankalpa.* As I have said, I generally prefer that a resolve be more specific and quantifiable, but "bears real fruit" had meaning for Patty, so that was the resolution with which she left the workshop.

Patty's *sankalpa* wound up bearing fruit in two stages. During the first stage, which lasted a few months, she became more mindful of being anxious. This may not sound particularly desirable, but because Patty managed to remain always mindful, it eventually dawned on her that her anxiety might have something to do with the fact that for nearly two decades she had dismissed her desire to paint. This realization may also have been helped by the fact that *kama*—the desire for the pleasure that beauty and art provide—was the desire toward which her unconscious had pointed her in the Bliss Meditation. But even though she recognized the possible link between her anxiety and not acting on her desire to paint, during those first few months she continued resisting and did nothing about her anxious feelings, perhaps because she had grown so accustomed to not responding to them.

Eventually the impulse to paint became stronger, however, and when resisting it became too much to bear, Patty enrolled in an art class. After just a few classes, her anxiety began to fade, and the second stage of her achieving her *sankalpa* soon unfolded. Not long after Patty started channeling her feelings into her art, it became apparent to everyone who saw her work that she was a remarkably talented artist. After less than a year of classes, her teacher encouraged her to participate in her first art show. I attended the opening and can tell you that her work was exceptional. She was the only one who was surprised to see all her paintings sell in just a few hours. One of those paintings now hangs in my home.

Patty managed to go a long way in her journey from being a person with a vague sense of anxiety to being a successful artist. However, the version of her story that I've just given you greatly oversimplifies her path to success; it was actually more of an odyssey, with setbacks, periods of self-doubt, and even a period when she stopped painting. The vital point that will emerge from the fuller version of the story is that Patty could not have achieved the change she did without first having taken certain key steps that helped her change her trajectory and allowed her to fulfill her destiny as a successful artist.

Until now, I've left out the critical piece of *how* Patty managed to get to her future as a painter. Surprisingly enough, the critical piece was sugar.

For years, Patty had eaten sugar compulsively, all day long. Her husband described her as a "sugar addict." An entire cupboard of their home was filled exclusively with bags of candy. Throughout the day, Patty would eat sweets, and if she felt worried and stressed, she would reach for more. In one sense, she was lucky, because she had a good metabolism and never gained much weight; but that also made her feel less urgency about breaking the habit, even though she knew it was an unhealthy one.

At the workshop, Patty realized her best chance of having a different and better future depended on having a powerful Departure Point. She made the bold decision to stop eating refined sugar completely. She threw out all the candy.

You can imagine that after years of using sugar to control her feelings, she initially had some rough times. Cravings for sugar would come up throughout the day, but instead of indulging them, she used them to her advantage. Whenever she felt a craving, she took a moment's pause and filled it with an affirmation of her *sankalpa*: "Always mindful of all my feelings and thoughts, the peace within me bears real fruit." In other words, in the clear and empty space she created with these pauses, which were quite frequent, she "seeded the gap," planting her intention ever deeper within herself. From the moment she began to practice doing this, her cravings became her leverage to change her trajectory. Deciding to give up her old habit was her Departure Point, and each of her cravings became an opportunity to "seed the gap" with her intention.

Very soon, Patty's cravings began to lessen and give way to a new confidence. She managed to go one month, then two, then three without any refined sugar. She lost fifteen pounds and started to feel and look better than she had in years. Most important, though, she was actively leveraging her impulse for sweets to chart a new and amazing life course. Having converted each call for sugar into a growing sense of making real and tangible progress toward her intention of "bearing fruit," she finally felt brave enough to enroll in an art class. That same feeling of courage enabled her to continue painting even while confronting various fears and self-limiting beliefs, particularly as they related to achieving success, and eventually gave her the courage to exhibit her art in public. She was becoming the painter, and the person, that she had always wanted to be.

> . . . .
> *Stillness is a more compelling force to influence and attract, and thereby help you fulfill your desires, than is desperation or even willpower alone.*
> . . . .

Today, Patty continues to paint and is a successful artist.

You, too, can disembark from your old trajectory and create new and powerful momentum toward fulfilling your *sankalpa* using the principle of the Departure Point and the technique of Seeding the Gap. Here's how.

CREATE YOUR DEPARTURE POINT, THEN SEED THE GAP

Step 1: Choosing a Habit to Give Up: Your Departure Point

The habit you are going to give up needs to be one that you deem nonconstructive and which you are prepared to let go. It also needs to be something you do on a regular basis, perhaps once or several times per day, or at least *think* about doing several times a day. It's best if the habit is a concrete action rather than a habit of thought, for the simple reason that it's easier to track whether or not you're doing something than to track whether or not you're thinking something.

For example, if the habit you choose to give up is smoking, it will be very easy to know if you have successfully given it up. On the other hand, if the habit you have chosen to give up is a particular negative thought, it will be harder to track whether or not you are successfully giving it up. You're either smoking or you're not, but you are thinking all day long and it's harder—not impossible, but more difficult—to follow each and every one of those thoughts and stop the negative ones.

To select the particular habit you are going to give up, you can refer to the list of bad or nonconstructive habits that I asked you to make at the end of Chapter Thirteen. After you've reviewed your list, if it occurs to you that a habit you may not have listed might be better leverage for a new direction in your life, by all means use that habit even though it's not on your list.

The habit you choose does not necessarily have to relate to the short-term goal toward which your *sankalpa* is directed. In other words, if your *sankalpa* is to exercise five times a week, you don't necessarily have to choose giving up the habit of watching television three or four hours per day. It may be useful to give it up, especially if you are aware that watching television is a distraction that makes it more difficult to exercise consistently, but the crucial thing is to choose a habit that has a strong enough hold on you that giving it up will be meaningful, regardless of whether or not it is obviously related to your intention or *sankalpa*.

It's also a good idea to know that giving it up is doable and that you're willing to give it up. Giving up a habit that is deeply ingrained and has a powerful sway over you will give you maximum leverage if you succeed—but if it's too hard, you may not. It's better to pick a habit that is not so challenging that you will fail to give it up. Sugar had a strong hold over Patty, but she felt that giving it up was doable, and she was willing to make the commitment.

You know best which habit will be the most effective for you to give up. Besides eating sweets, examples of habits that students have successfully given up include fingernail biting, cracking knuckles, gossiping, and many different kinds of overindulgence—high-fat foods, coffee, soda, wine, shopping sprees, surfing the Internet, listening to talk radio, watching late-night television, work, and so on.

Step 2: Using Your Departure Point to Seed the Gap

After you have decided which habit you are going to give up as your Departure Point, here's how the Seeding the Gap method works.

1. At some point in the day, you will have an impulse to engage in your habit.

2. Rather than satisfy the impulse, stop.

3. At this instant, turn your attention away from your impulse to engage in the habit and toward a Higher Source: an inner source of peace and calm, an infinite intelligence outside of you, God, Nature, or even a remembrance of the love and support of people to whom you are closest.

4. For an instant, rest in this experience. Relax. Surrender into it. Be nowhere other than right there.

5. Now, mindful of that experience of your Higher Source, recall your *sankalpa*. Mentally repeat the precise words while you remember the feeling as well as the image you associate with it. With full feeling and knowledge, have the certainty and confidence that your intention has already been fulfilled.

6. Give thanks.

This is the entire process of Seeding the Gap. Its six steps should take you less than a minute and can be done anytime, any place, and whether you're alone or not, because no one ever has to know you're doing it. Simply repeat the steps each time you find yourself thinking about or craving the habit you've chosen to give up. It is ideal to do this a minimum of once or twice each day, more often if the impulse toward your habit comes up more often. There may be no more accessible or far-reaching method for creating new and powerful momentum toward achieving an intention.

At a certain point, whichever habit you choose to work with may no longer provide the leverage it once did. In Patty's case, the first month of giving up sugar was much harder than months three, four, or five, but by then she had created a new trajectory with its own momentum that was leading her to her goal.

It's vital that the habit you choose to give up generates real momentum toward your own version of that same place. If and when the habit you've chosen is no longer providing you with sufficient leverage, you'll want to pick another one to work with until you feel that you have really moved your momentum in the direction of achieving your *sankalpa*.

Simple as it is, the technique of Seeding the Gap is very empowering because it makes you increasingly capable of achieving your goals. Its effects are twofold. First, it helps you break free of the negative pull of your past, which means that it is reducing the resistance side of the Creation Equation. Second, it propels you toward your goal by allowing you to connect to a force greater than yourself, which makes achieving your intention all the more likely.

Let's look at both of these effects more closely.

When you pause to establish a clear and empty state of mind, this "gap" is, by definition, free from the distortion of your unconscious, where doubts, contrary beliefs, and misapprehensions of all kinds are stored. This silent, reflective space is an ever-present link to sacred and sublime intelligence or Source. While you are resting in it, if only during a slight pause, your intention is to reestablish your connection to a place that is boundless, infinite in possibility, and free from all the unconscious "stuff" that would otherwise obstruct you from achieving your goal.

This point is essential. From the tantric perspective, stillness, coupled with expanded awareness, is by far the most powerful medium by which your desire can affect your destiny. I conveyed this idea earlier, when describing the fourth intensity of desire, manifestation, and again in my description of Relax into Greatness. But it's worth emphasizing again that stillness is a more compelling force to influence and attract, and thereby to help you fulfill your desires, than is desperation or even willpower alone.

CHAPTER 16

· · · ·

HOW INTENTION FLOWERS INTO FULFILLMENT

Stephanie needed a breakthrough. After a recent divorce and a bad investment decision, she found herself working sixty to seventy hours a week just to meet the mortgage payments on the two houses she owned. A monstrous downturn in the real estate market had only made matters worse. The house she had bought as an "investment" had been on the market for two years and home sales in the city in which she lived were at a standstill; property values were in a steep decline.

Stephanie wasn't trying to make a killing in real estate, just hoping to get more balance in her life. To do this, she needed to sell at least one of her two properties. She had been repeating her intention—"The Lakewood home sold and we are out of debt"—with no success. She realized she needed a Departure Point—something, anything, to change her momentum.

She determined her most immediate and accessible Departure Point would be to stop constantly checking her e-mail. It may not sound like much, but for Stephanie checking e-mail had become a compulsion. From the time she got up in the morning till just before going to sleep, every five or ten minutes she'd look to see if anything new had come into her in-box. To leverage her way toward change, Stephanie decided she would check her personal e-mail only twice a day, once before work and once after.

The first few weeks were a real challenge for Stephanie, both at work and at home. During the first week, she would often find herself reading several e-mails, then surfing the Internet, then returning to her in-box to check for new e-mails before she even realized what she was doing. However, each time she did stop herself from indulging in her old habit and made herself pause long enough to do the Seeding the Gap exercise, it gave her the sense that she was taking charge of her life. And every time that happened, she felt a wave of energy and strength—even a sense of victory.

Day by day, Stephanie stopped herself more frequently. Sometime during the second week, she had an insight. Ever since her childhood, she'd kept herself busy, occupying herself with even the most trivial things as a way to avoid feeling vulnerable. Checking e-mail was just one more way of staying busy, and she realized that it was keeping her stuck in the past. When ten days had passed and she felt that she had broken her e-mail habit, she was elated, assuming that she was over it.

A few days later, however, she found herself lost again in her old habit. Every time she compulsively checked her e-mail, she felt a tinge of sadness and guilt, but she did it nonetheless. Amazed that her habit seemed to have more power over her than she did over it, Stephanie resolved a few weeks later to get on the right side of it once and for all.

Her determination was fueled by her realization that her general compulsion "to do" was distancing her from living and from pursuing the deeper meaning and purpose of her life. She saw that while the habit of staying perpetually busy was a strategy that had been effective during her unhappy childhood, it was no longer serving her best interests. She could now sense that it was keeping her bound to experiences and feelings that she had outgrown. That was why each time she chose not to indulge her compulsion to check her e-mail, she'd experience a surge of inner power—the energy released by freeing herself from the chains of the past. As soon as she became committed to breaking the habit once and for all, she felt freer, more expansive, and less the victim of her life's circumstances.

Putting the brakes on her habit became a welcome opportunity to use the Seeding the Gap method to open herself to higher forces and repeat her *sankalpa*. She did this several times throughout the day and evening—each time she had the impulse to check her e-mail. Then, out of nowhere, it happened! A couple of months after creating her Departure Point, an offer came in and Stephanie sold her house. There are several plausible explanations, but what we do know for sure is that the real estate market didn't change even though Stephanie's fate did.

The Power of Directed Thought

Research in quantum physics and the related field of string theory has helped establish a scientific basis for some of the ancient teachings about how the mind's reach, depending on the clarity of your mind and thoughts, is potentially limitless.

Pioneers such as Niels Bohr, Max Planck, Albert Einstein, and the quantum physicists who succeeded them helped shift the Western view of the world we live in. Your five senses may be telling you that the book you are reading is distinct from the hands holding it, which are distinct from the chair in which you are sitting or the bed on which you are lying, which is distinct from the office or home you are in, which is distinct from the world outside—but your senses are deceiving you. $E = MC^2$, Einstein's groundbreaking theory, tells us that matter and energy are essentially two different forms of the same thing. The universe we live in is energy—what yogis call *prana*—trapped in material form. Both Einstein and the ancient sages taught that at a subtle level the world and everything in it is essentially *pranic,* composed of energy and intelligence.

Once you accept the physical stuff of our world as a manifestation of a vibrant pool of energy and intelligence, it's not a giant leap to imagine that thought is just another form of energy and thus can and does influence everything around it. The idea that energy follows thought, a tantric teaching that an increasing amount of scientific research by quantum physicists is helping to prove, explains how attitude can affect your health and how, as my teacher Mani would often assert, "each thought wave influences the mind and therein affects your destiny."

When those thoughts are powerful enough, they become manifest. This is evident in the study I mentioned earlier, which found that women at a fertility clinic who were prayed for became pregnant at twice the rate of those who were not prayed for. The prayers (a form of thought) had a tangible effect on the world of matter. Perhaps, too, Stephanie's work to seed the gap and solidify her Departure Point helped effect change. The more potent your thoughts, the more likely it is you will be able to generate real, material changes in the world. This raises the question of how to make your thoughts more powerful. To understand how, at least from the view of the ancient tradition, we turn to a description of the mind, which throughout Vedic wisdom is referred to metaphorically as a body of water.

> . . . .
> "Creation is only the projection into form of that which already exists."
> —SRIMAD BHAGAVATAM
> . . . .

Intentions, like all other forms of thought, are waves that silently ripple, expanding out from the mind to the universe. When the mind that is generating an intention is quiet and centered, the ripple expands outward from that center, sending a signal that is free of distortion and disturbance. Transmitting your intention from the calm of prayer or meditation endows that intention with the most power and thus allows you to have the most influence on the material world. An intention that originates from a less than quiet mind will not be as clearly transmitted to the universe and thus will be a less potent manifesting force.

To effect real change, an intention needs to touch the invisible, all-pervading world of *prana* or life force. Conveying your intention when your mind is clear magnifies its reach; in other words, the depth of your sense of ease or stillness will determine the power of your intention and its potential for fulfillment. This is how the ancient tradition looks upon what are commonly called miracles—it is how Jesus Christ could manifest his intention to feed thousands through the miracle of loaves and bring Lazarus back from the dead, and how Bengali Baba was able to resurrect the prince of Bhawal from the dead. Jesus and Bengali Baba could perform such miracles because of their utter and complete connection to the Father or Source of all things.

I'm not suggesting that any of us can rise to the level of spiritual illumination of Jesus or Bengali Baba. But each of us is capable of the kind of stillness involved in Seeding the Gap. To the extent that your intentions are seeded in the auspiciousness of silence and complete ease, you can be certain that your *sankalpa* will become a more potent force and move you closer to your goal as well as your goal closer to you.

Quantum theory gives us the scientific explanation for how thought can affect the future. Quantum physicists hold that all matter consists of waves of pulsing light; each infinitesimally small burst is called a quantum. In the vast field of pulsing light and intelligence, there are no boundaries between material and non-material reality and between past, future, and present. This principle provides the basis of how the ancient tradition explains how thought (non-material reality) can effect "real" changes in our material world. "Creation is only the projection into form of that which already exists," the *Srimad Bhagavatam* tells us. In other words, whatever you are hoping for—whether it is the life of your dreams, a positive change in the world we live in, healing, or enlightenment—already exists. Depending on where you place attention and the quality of your awareness as you are doing so, you increase or decrease the likelihood of it becoming a tangible reality. That is why taking a pause to clear your mind each time you plant your intention is so powerful, and how Stephanie, using the Seeding the Gap technique, could achieve her desire.

There is another explanation as to how Seeding the Gap could have led Stephanie and countless others with whom I've worked to fulfill their *sankalpas*. This one draws on neither the ancient teachings of yoga nor the latest findings of theoretical physics (though it is compatible with both). It says, quite simply, that the reason Stephanie was able to defy the odds and sell her home was because she changed. By letting go of a habit (her Departure Point) and being willing to walk through the challenges of doing so, she set in motion a sequence of changes that allowed her to achieve her desire. Although subtle at first, these shifts gradually built and created a ripple effect of enough significance that it changed her future.

As I've said, not long after beginning the process of stopping her old pattern of checking her e-mail multiple times per hour, Stephanie became more conscious of both her habit and herself. Almost immediately after stopping it, she began to feel more positive; in subtle ways, Stephanie began to act differently. She felt different as she spoke to others. She felt freer, with more choices; she carried herself differently, and as the effects of the practice accumulated, her outlook on life continued to improve. Her commitment to continue practicing Relax into Greatness helped to empower her to change. Every time she did the exercise, she experienced herself as having already achieved her desire, and this increased her sense of ease. She hadn't deliberately set out to change, it was simply the by-product of practicing Seeding the Gap along with Relax into Greatness.

A new, more authentic version of Stephanie was taking shape. And given the extent of Stephanie's internal changes, every one of her interactions with other people was different. In short, the whole of Stephanie's life might have become just different enough to tip the scales in her favor. After she chose her Departure Point and started to work with Seeding the Gap, while continuing to practice Relax into Greatness, everything she was doing and thinking had repercussions that ultimately delivered a buyer to her.

Does this sound realistic, or does it seem as mystical as the teachings of tantra, as intangible as the world of quantum physics? Of course, another possible explanation for Stephanie selling her house, or for anybody achieving any intention, is coincidence—it just happened to happen. But I hope that by now you are open to other possibilities.

I believe that there may be no single teaching in *The Four Desires* that could prove more instrumental to your ability to successfully negotiate the terrain that stands between you and the achievement of your *sankalpa* than this: the slightest change in the quality of your actions, attitude, or timing can make all the difference as to whether you will be in the right place at the right time to fulfill the destiny you seek.

Examining how intention may influence the material world and how it can help us achieve our desires places us at the heart of the mystery of how destiny unfolds, facing some of life's most enduring questions: Can mortal beings actually shape the future? If so, to what extent? What are the relationships between fate and faith, present and future? We've answered some of these questions at least in part. The Vedic tradition offers us additional answers and additional knowledge. Let's turn to it so that we can make the journey of fulfilling our destiny less of a mystery and more easily navigable.

Improving the Odds

The story of how I met my teacher Mani is the perfect illustration of how destiny unfolds. The year was 1980; I was twenty-two and had gone out dancing with some friends—a rather unlikely scenario for eventually meeting one's spiritual teacher. I was in a nightclub filled to capacity when I noticed a tall, attractive blonde across the dance floor and made my way over to her. Soon after I said hello, it became clear she was not interested. A few hours later, I approached her again, but rather than press the issue I began talking to her friend, Rena, in case the blonde might have a change of heart. After a few minutes, I learned that Rena and I had something in common: we had both started yoga about twelve months earlier. I was very eager to move forward in my yoga practice, and what Rena told me about her classes intrigued me. Before the evening was over, Rena and I agreed that the following week we would take each other to our respective yoga classes. I asked for her number, but rather than give it to me, she asked for mine, which I gave to her. She said she'd call before the weekend, so I left that night without any details about the location of her yoga class or even the name of her teacher.

Two weeks went by with no call. But as destiny—or luck; call it what you will—would have it, I ran into her soon thereafter in the tea section of the local health food store. More than a little embarrassed, she said, "I'm so sorry. I meant to call you. . . . I would have called you. . . . I got so busy. . . . I will call you. I promise I will call you. Yes, I do have your number. Don't worry; I will call." She seemed genuine. I expected to hear from her.

Another two weeks went by with no call. Then I ran into her again. This time it was on a Saturday, surrounded by thousands of people on the boardwalk near the beach. It was an odd feeling to stand in the midst of a throng face-to-face with someone and know that I was the last person she wanted or expected to see. Rena didn't say it, but I could see from the look on her face that she was thinking, *What are the odds?* Again, she apologized: "I'm so sorry, I've just been really busy. I've been meaning to call you. I promise I will call you. I can't wait to go to your yoga class." Despite her sincere tone, I was now somewhat skeptical that she would ever call me, and—no surprise—she didn't.

But three weeks later, just as I was walking into a restaurant, who should walk out? "Oh my God," she said in amazement, "I guess I *really am* supposed to call you." This time she did.

Less than a week later, Rena came to my yoga class and I went to hers, where I met Alan Finger. Within a week, I began studying with him regularly, practicing yoga and meditation. A few months later, I met his father, Mani, whose presence, wisdom, and erudition captured my ear and heart. Soon Mani, with the help of Alan, would become my guiding light into the ancient traditions of the Vedas and tantra. For the next seventeen years, my intensive studies with the two of them would change my life forever and would become my foundation as a teacher, as a man, and as author of the book you are reading.

It's worth noting that all of these "chance" encounters took place in Los Angeles, a city of more than twelve million people spread out over many miles, where you often have to go to great pains to see the people you *do* know. Granted, Rena and I did have nightclubs, yoga, and health food in common, but that cannot explain how or why our paths would cross four different times within just a few weeks.

As improbable and seemingly remote as the events were that led me to my teachers, there's nothing particularly uncommon about it in regard to the way that destiny unfolds in our lives. To prove the point, I usually ask at least one participant in my seminars to share the sequence of events that led them to meet his or her loved one or the links in the chain that led the person to study with me or to attend the seminar. The stories I hear are usually no less improbable or seemingly remote than the story of how I met Mani.

On close examination, most people's destinies seem to hinge on some random meeting or encounter. Reflect for a moment on how your parents met, or consider the links in the chain that led you to the person you married or to your business partner, the career you chose, or even to the city you live in. What one or two "chance" encounters have been the most influential in your life? What led you to this book? How many things had to happen or people did you have to meet in order for you to be reading these words? Viewed objectively, what were the odds?

So it happens that an incidental encounter can become the pivot around which your life changes forever—for better or, sometimes, for worse. This means that your future—and, more to the point, fulfilling your intention or *sankalpa*—often turns on little more than being in a particular place at a particular time.

I understand that some readers might not subscribe to the idea that we can have an influence on externally oriented events, such as Stephanie's selling her house or my meeting my teachers. It's possible to argue that these stories illustrate the workings of pure coincidence and that life is shaped by nothing but chance. This worldview holds that there is no organizing principle and no inherent meaning that connects a human being to the unfolding of events in his or her life. There is no purpose in what has happened or will happen.

A second argument assumes that destiny is predetermined. I was supposed to meet Mani and become a yoga teacher. Thus the blonde in the nightclub, who led me to her friend Rena, who after multiple chance encounters took me to her yoga class, which was taught by Alan Finger—all were just links in a chain leading me to an already determined outcome.

There is a third option that suggests that the fate of our world and everything in it is to some degree fluid, the result of some combination of chance and predetermination. This line of thought describes the principle that there are many possible outcomes; some are fixed and will happen, others are likely to occur, and the rest are little more than dormant possibilities that remain so until something activates them. By extension this means that we can have a role in determining our destiny. The tantric tradition views the unfolding of destiny according to this third option. It begins with the premise that each of us possesses varying degrees of capacity as a co-creator of our destiny, both individual and collective, and suggests that this capacity can be increased—which is why tantra has developed a systematic approach to manifesting intention.

From the Vedic and tantric perspectives, there are no coincidences or chance encounters; everything is based on cause and effect. Thus, based on some cause, a part of me—let's call it my psyche, where the unconscious and the soul meet—placed me in each of those situations. In other words, in order for that fourth and finally fruitful meeting with Rena to take place, my psyche arranged for me to walk down the street and open the door of that restaurant at precisely the right moment.

To take this a step further, since my encounters with Rena did not take place in a vacuum, my psyche was able to navigate through an infinitely large and complex array of possibilities. To meet her in each of the locations at the precise time that she was there, I had to encounter just the right number of red and green lights and find just the right parking space (if I had had to park even a block farther away from the health food store, the boardwalk, or the restaurant, everything might have been different). I even needed to have the right number of distractions and phone calls occupying my day prior to getting in my car and driving to the restaurant where that fourth meeting was to occur.

> . . . .
>
> *The slightest change in the quality of your actions, attitude, or timing can make all the difference as to whether or not you will be in the right place at the right time to fulfill the destiny you seek.*
>
> . . . .

This intuitive part of me was able to create a sequence where time and place converged to create an auspicious outcome (a phenomenon often called *synchronicity*). All of this was completely beyond the scope and capabilities of my conscious mind; indeed, my conscious mind could never have orchestrated it even if it knew what it should be looking for. What the conscious mind *can* do, as we've seen, is to plant a conscious intention in the psyche. This is the basis of the tantric science of affecting destiny: to methodically seed your intention in the psyche, which can then lead you to achieve your goal.

At the time I met Rena, I had already planted the conscious intention of mastering yoga. But at no time was I consciously looking for Rena, or for the teacher I did not know I wanted. When Rena and I finally ran into each other at the restaurant, I was simply following an impulse to have lunch at that particular place at that particular time. One minute earlier or later and our paths would not have crossed and I might not ever have met my future teacher.

Throughout the course of your life, your psyche, holding the causes or seeds of your past, leads you through myriad events, which (unless and until your psyche is programmed to do otherwise), will lead you to a predetermined fate. It does this by responding to your deepest, most powerful desires and putting you in exactly the right circumstances in which those desires, regardless of whether they are in alignment with your conscious desires, can be materialized.

The implications of this are, as we learned when we looked at *vikalpa* (contrary deepest driving desires) as a force of resistance, that if you are to achieve your conscious desires—desires that are *not* predetermined— you first need to solicit the help of your unconscious. You can do this by properly planting your conscious desires into the unconscious through Relax into Greatness. And by using the Departure Point and Seeding the Gap techniques, you generate even more momentum toward achieving the future to which both you and your soul aspire.

Once your intention is deeply planted within the unconscious, you need to be able to hear where your intuition is guiding you. The final, critical piece is then acting on what you have heard. *Action in response to intuition connects you to the links in the chain of causality that lead to the manifestation of your intention.*

To the extent that you become masterful at knowing what to do and then doing what you know, you increase your ability to make the Creation Equation work in your favor. We'll begin our exploration of this final element in the Creation Equation with a discussion of how to awaken your power to know what to do.

CHAPTER 17

. . . .

THE POWER TO *KNOW* WHAT TO DO

Alone in her apartment, Kristin had been thinking all morning of something I'd said to her six months earlier. "Kristin, I'm not going to tell you what I think you should do, because you need to learn to rely on your judgment. The more content you feel, the clearer your judgment will be. So what I *am* going to do is give you a meditation practice that will help you build your sense of self-worth and link you to your natural state of joy and inspiration. If you're established in that state, it will be easier to know what to do and trust yourself to make the right decisions about what's best for you and your daughter."

After months of avoiding it, Kristin gathered herself and finally sat down to meditate. For the past three years, she had meditated fairly regularly, but in the last six months she had had so many things to do and so much on her mind that the prospect of sitting still seemed intolerable. She was doing it now because she felt fearful and desperately in need of what meditation used to give her.

Within moments of closing her eyes, her mind had already raced in a thousand directions, which only added to her irritation. Not only was she distracted, she felt like a frustrated beginner all over again. "Slow down my thoughts? Impossible . . . All I am doing is thinking. . . . That was a thought. . . . And that was another. . . . I'm a mess. . . . I must be kidding myself. . . . How the hell did I ever do this?" Kristin concluded that this was going to be another exercise in futility, but she carried on anyway, thinking, "What the heck? Just keeping my body still for the next twenty minutes will be a kind of victory." She told herself to focus on her meditation and just let "whatever is going to happen, happen."

Moments later, as Kristin's mind became more focused, the loud street sounds below her apartment began to fade. Her body relaxed as once again she recalled my words: "your natural state of joy and inspiration." Then it was as if something pulled her deeper into meditation. Slowly she was finding it easier to focus her attention.

As Kristin realized she was thinking less and feeling more, she became aware of what she later described to me as a "presence," a feeling of aliveness that was greater than the sum of her parts. Just then, a thought surfaced: "I've never been this deep before. *This* is why people meditate." The thought quickly disappeared and she felt herself approaching an even deeper state of stillness.

Kristin was being drawn into the very thing that has inspired and transformed the lives of meditators from time immemorial. As the mind gets quiet, we gain access to worlds hidden from ordinary perception. We enter a realm far beyond the ups and downs of everyday life, and there we eventually discover an endless source of inspiration, healing, and wisdom.

Kristin now found herself resting in utter contentment and just self-aware enough to silently delight in it. As if she had uncovered something incredibly precious, she did her best to hold on to it, all the while knowing that wanting it too much would probably make it vanish. But rather than fade, the feeling grew!

Moments later, she was in awe, feeling surrounded by what she felt was love; she was ecstatic. A ripple of thought passed through her: "I couldn't possibly feel better than I feel right at this moment." Then a part of her realized that she could relax even *more* deeply. Suddenly everything went absolutely quiet. She rested in this place for what could have been twenty seconds or twenty minutes. It was impossible to know.

Then, just as suddenly, Kristin experienced a sense of vibrancy in every cell of her body; her spine effortlessly grew taller. She felt utterly alert and wholly at ease. As this feeling grew, she became aware of a kind of light-filled presence, and with it came the feeling that a doorway to intuition had suddenly opened. More than at any other time in her life, she felt complete and trusting of herself and her capacities, certain that this light knew exactly what she needed to know. At that instant she felt a surge of intuition, a gut feeling that told her, "If you want love and to feel safe, stop. You need to move on. Once and for all, let go! If not for you, you need to leave for *her*. The two of you will be fine, better than fine."

Kristin knew "her" was Kira, her daughter, the thought of whom seemed to flip a switch. As if Kristin was watching a movie, memories flashed before her: getting pregnant, marriage, giving birth. Shortly thereafter she saw the beginning of all the troubles: her husband pulling away, spending less time at home, becoming increasingly remote as both husband and father; Kristin crying herself to sleep, left to wonder if he was coming home; Kira asleep next to her. He was having an affair. He blamed her. Arguments grew louder; he'd disappear for days to "stay with friends." Each time he returned she'd beg him to work with her on saving their marriage.

Kristin longed to give her daughter exactly what she had never had: a stable home with two loving parents. She couldn't envision leaving Kira's father, the only man she'd ever loved, or living alone, raising their daughter by herself. No matter how bad things got, no matter how often those who really cared about her told her she should leave, she couldn't face it. She felt trapped. She hated her life, hated what she had become. That was how she'd spent the past five years.

Kristin's eyes were still closed as the movie reel came to an end. Her meditative experience of a few minutes ago was a distant memory. Then she remembered: today she was helping her husband move back in. It was what she wanted, right? Now she wasn't so sure. The voice had told her to "let go." It dawned on her—for the first time ever—that she could leave and everything would "be fine, better than fine." Really?

She flashed back to something we had talked about the last time she and I met. "Perhaps, Kristin," I'd told her, "the reason you don't feel as uncomfortable as you should with the way your husband treats you is because you've spent so much of your life in pain. Over time, it's become so familiar that it's more comfortable for you to be in pain."

I then shared with her an analogy I had never used in a personal consultation before and have never used since: "Put a frog in a pot of room-temperature water and turn up the heat. Because the rise of temperature is gradual, the frog remains acclimated. It isn't uncomfortable until it's too late. At that point, the frog is cooked. On the other hand, drop a frog in a pot of water that's already boiling and it leaps out. Starting with your childhood, Kristin, you've been in a pot of water with the temperature slowly rising. The people who truly care about you look at your life and think, 'My God, the water's boiling. Why doesn't she jump out of the pot?' "

A little more than twenty-four hours later, Kristin sent me this e-mail:

Dear Rod,

I am excited to share with you all that has come about for me. To make a really long and unnecessary story short . . . The frog jumped out of the water.

It wasn't hard. It didn't hurt!

Kristin

Kristin came out of meditation knowing that she had to end her marriage. Why—or better yet, *how*—did she suddenly have the insight to know and the courage to do what was best for her? Through meditation she was able to tap into both her intuition and her ability to act on it. "We are safe and loved" was her *sankalpa*. Through meditation she suddenly saw a path to fulfilling her *sankalpa* that she had never seen before. She now knew that she could be a sufficient source of love and safety for Kira as well as for herself.

One of the underlying teachings of the Bhagavad Gita is that the purpose of yoga is to make the unconscious conscious. It may occur to you to ask why anyone would want to do this, especially if you are under the impression that the unconscious is little more than an endless supply of repressed memories and self-defeating beliefs. The answer is that the yoga tradition teaches that this is only part of the story, that the unconscious includes *everything* you are not aware of, not just the negative material but some things that are wholly positive. The stuff with which you eventually make creative leaps is waiting in your unconscious. Indeed, according to the yoga tradition, a clear vision of ultimate reality resides in your unconscious. When you awaken spiritually, that understanding becomes conscious. Thus, since the beginning of time, yogis, saints, and seers of all faiths have deliberately waded into their unconscious in order first to understand themselves completely and express what is best of themselves, then eventually to discover God and the mysteries of the universe.

But how do we gain access to the riches within? The answer is found in the one thing that most, if not all, spiritual traditions (including the

Vedas, Christianity, Islam, tantra, and Buddhism) agree upon: the power of silence. Silence is indeed golden.

We live in a world that is constantly in flux. Remember that under normal circumstances your mind, whose charge it is to perceive and make sense of this world of change and uncertainty, is itself part of this constant change, ceaselessly moving from one thought to the next. The result, as Paramahansa Yogananda once wrote, is that "God's plan for us often becomes obscured by the conflicts of human life and so we lose the inner guidance that would save us from chasms of misery." Once you are able to quiet the mind, as Kristin did on the day she came out of her meditation knowing that she had to leave her husband, you stand at the threshold of timeless wisdom, the inner teacher that is your soul.

. . . .

Yogis, saints, and seers of all faiths have deliberately waded into their unconscious . . . to understand themselves completely and express what is best of themselves.

. . . .

According to the yoga tradition, the thing that sparked Kristin's transformation and allowed her to begin a new chapter in her life was a glimpse of her soul's light or wisdom. This light is ever-present, yet all too often it goes unrecognized. It is the guiding force that dwells within each person and empowers us to see and act in a way that is free from conditioning and everything that holds us back—self-defeating beliefs, negative patterns, psychological baggage, self-esteem issues, the limiting influences of family and culture. The morning Kristin finally sat down to meditate again, she experienced that guiding presence; doing so set wheels into motion that would change her life and her daughter's for the better, forever.

It's not wishful thinking to say that we each have access to divine or heavenly guidance ad infinitum. This is a teaching that comes right out of the ancient texts and is a central theme of the Bhagavad Gita. I believe it is one of the ancient tradition's most inspiring and life-affirming messages.

According to Vedic wisdom, we are each born with a blueprint to achieve a full and contented life. Your soul holds that blueprint, and the higher aspects of your mind—namely, your intuition or conscience—are the means by which you can read that blueprint and let it guide you to

fulfill its master plan. In the *Yoga Sutras,* the defining text of the yoga tradition written by the great sage Patanjali, we find the following teaching:
"By mastering *samyama* [meditation and its various stages] *prajna*
dawns." *Prajna* is commonly translated as "the light of wisdom." All of us
can experience the light of wisdom.

Another Sanskrit term for this illumined wisdom is *dhi. Dhi* is intrinsic awareness, what is sometimes called a "gut feeling" or "knowingness." It is, in essence, conscience, but conscience with a broader
meaning than the one we give the word in our everyday conversations.
Dhi is more than our personal barometer or inner voice of morality—
more than what helps us distinguish right from wrong. In the context of
the ancient tradition, *dhi* refers to the higher aspect of the mind. It is the
inner voice of higher wisdom that knows and is capable of guiding you
to do precisely the right thing at precisely the right time. In effect, *dhi* is
the light of the inner teacher that dwells within you. Intuition is your
way of hearing it.

Dhi is the knowingness that always understands what actions are
going to help you thrive and what actions are not. Again, whether you
consciously hear it or not, some part of you always *knows.* For every question, a part of you is ready with the answer and a clear direction for what
you need to know and do.

Whether you practice yoga or not, you possess that inner knowingness; you have that voice. I have heard it tell me to stop working and
spend some time in Nature; other times it tells me to rest, tickle my kids, or make a date with my wife, Gina. It tells me to be grateful. It told me to move to Colorado. It has even told me to put more money in the parking meter. Without fail, it keeps telling me to practice meditation daily, eat well, exercise, and be gentle with Nature.

We are each born with a blueprint to achieve a full and contented life. Your soul holds that blueprint, and the higher aspects of your mind are the means by which you can read that blueprint and let it guide you to fulfill its master plan.

Masaru Ibuka, co-founder and chair-
man of Sony, lived his life guided by this voice. Whenever he had an important choice to make, one that would affect his future or that of his multinational corpora-
tion, he would turn to his intuition for the final word. After researching
sales reports, hearing from consultants, and reviewing marketing trends,

Ibuka would withdraw and have his assistant prepare a traditional Japanese tea ceremony.

The tea ceremony is a precise ritual, performed the same way each time. It invokes a reflective and tranquil atmosphere. Watching as well as doing it is a form of meditation. Once the tea was prepared, Ibuka would hold a cupful while silently posing a yes-or-no question. He would then take a sip of tea and listen, carefully observing how his body responded and how the tea felt in his stomach. If it felt good, he interpreted that as a yes; if it didn't, it was a no. "I trust my gut, and I know how it works," he said. "My mind is not that smart, but my body is." What he heard and what shaped many of the decisions that led to his company's astounding success were found by tapping into *dhi*.

Masaru Ibuka is not the only king of industry who relied on intuition. Ray Kroc bought the first McDonald's when he couldn't afford it but had a really good hunch. As he put it, "My funny bone instinct kept urging me on." Conrad Hilton, founder of the Hilton chain of hotels, used his intuition to bid on the world's largest hotel and ended up the successful bidder by a margin of only $200. He said, "I know when I have a problem and have done all I can: thinking, figuring, planning, I keep listening in a sort of inside silence until something clicks and I feel a right answer."

The voice is ever-present and never wrong about leading you to what is right for you. As we've seen, the key to the future you seek may be as simple as making sure

> . . . .
>
> *For intuition to grow as a force in your life, you have to learn to honor it.*
>
> . . . .

that you are in front of the right door opening at the right time, and the best way to increase the likelihood of being there is to let *dhi* be your guide. While everyone possesses *dhi*, some are more sensitive to it than others. However, it is within everyone's grasp to *learn* to hear it. You can easily train yourself to tap into it and allow it to guide you, the same way that Kristin did. The process for tuning into *dhi* begins with stilling your mind, which is the purpose of the Healing the Heart Meditation, described below. Learning to still your mind does not require you to become a master of meditation. However, the more often you practice meditation, the easier it will become to access that inner silence and the wisdom that issues from it. In time and with practice, the voice of *dhi* will become stronger and clearer, and to the extent that you respond to it, you will find yourself more and more in the right place at the right time, doing the right thing. As the great teacher and sage Swami Satyananda Saraswati once wrote, "When you develop true sensitivity the whole world will be an open book to you, revealing on each page new secrets and wonderful knowledge."

The Technique for Accessing Your *Dhi*, which I walk you through at the end of this chapter, after the Healing the Heart Meditation, is a systematic process to tap into your voice of knowingness. It can be used whenever you have a question or seek guidance about how to achieve your *sankalpa* or make any other important decision. The key is to approach *dhi* less by trying to reach for answers than by trusting that they are already within you, just waiting to be recognized.

Before starting, here are some tips on the right way to ask questions:

- Develop your skill gradually by starting out with simpler questions, not life-defining ones.
- To hone your skill at asking precise, clear questions, it's a good idea to start with yes/no questions.
- To learn how to listen, you may even want to start with questions to which you already know the answers (for example, "Should I overeat today?").
- Make sure the way you phrase the question addresses exactly what you want to know. It can be helpful to write it down beforehand and refine it, until you feel sure that the question is specific enough. If your question is vague, your answer may also be vague, and less than helpful.
- Start from a place of "no-thing-ness." Silence is the abode of intuition. Be certain that, at some level, you can feel silence before you ask your question.
- Be open. Trust that a response will come. Remember, for every question there is an answer—the very part of you that has asked the question is ready with the answer.

Here's some advice about listening for answers:

- The way you will sense your inner voice of wisdom or guidance depends to a large degree on how you learn—
whether your primary aptitude is auditory, visual, or
kinesthetic. If you are more of an auditory learner, you will
be more likely to access intuition by hearing it. If you are
more visual, you will most likely see it in some way. If you
are more kinesthetic, you will feel it as sensation in your
body.

- The response may be a word, short phrase, or sentence.
Or it may be little more than a subtle sensation. (That was
all Masaru Ibuka relied on for his answers.) If, after posing
your question, you feel a quiet vibrancy or light-filled feeling, consider that a yes. If you feel a dark and dense sensation, your answer should be considered a no.

- When wisdom speaks, it often conveys something you
don't know or expect. Nothing mutes that voice more than
expectations or hope (that's the reason for Step 3, releasing expectations and needs). The more unattached to results you are, the more fully that voice can express itself to
you as you listen. The more relaxed you are emotionally
and physically, the more wondrously the process will unfold.

- Especially in the early stages of practicing accessing your
dhi, it's possible that the first answer to your question that
you perceive will not be from your *dhi*. Often it will be your
conscious mind giving you what it thinks is the right response, and the answer it delivers can get in the way of
your *dhi*, obscuring your inner guidance. (Be cautious
about answers that go on and on. More than likely, such a
response means that it's your rational mind speaking,
rather than your inner guidance.)

- Sometimes you may have to wait for a second or even a
third response before you get one that comes from your
dhi. In time and with practice, you will be able to access
dhi much more directly and quickly.

Healing the Heart Meditation

Stillness is the seat of intuition, where it begins and ends. Deep calm and ease are the state that allows you to move beyond the limitation of your rational mind. This is why the first step in accessing your *dhi* is meditation. A regular meditation practice is invaluable. If you do not already have a meditation practice, I recommend that you use any of the meditations in this book on a regular basis.

I chose the Healing the Heart Meditation to give to Kristin because, if practiced regularly, it leads to increased emotional balance, self-confidence, and self-reliance. If you prefer to use another meditation technique to lead into the *dhi* exercise, simply substitute it for the Healing the Heart Meditation.

The Sanskrit name of the heart center is *anahata,* which means, "unstruck" or "the place where no sorrow can enter." An ancient scripture states, "Joy permanently resides in our heart." Another teaching describes that there is a light in the heart that is "beyond all sorrow." The heart these teachings are referring to is the spiritual heart, the one in the center of your chest. Whether or not we see it, even in our darkest hours, joy is there, always.

The Healing the Heart Meditation releases sadness, emotional pain, and suffering and helps you reestablish your connection to joy. The basis of the technique is letting go of false ideas and negative feelings in favor of absorbing and identifying with this inner joy—your source of universal love and light.

You can record the instructions for the Healing the Heart Meditation and for the Technique for Accessing Your *Dhi* and play them for yourself to guide you through the steps, or you can get the CD at www.rodstryker.com.

HEALING THE HEART MEDITATION PRACTICE

Sit tall. Close your eyes and completely relax. Become aware of your body. . . . Take a moment to scan it. Starting at the top of your head, have the intention to deeply relax. Relax your scalp . . . forehead . . . and face . . . relax the back of your head . . . relax the neck . . . and throat . . . relax your shoulders . . . upper back . . . and chest or breast area. . . . relax your heart. For a moment become aware of your heartbeat. Have the intention to hear your heart beat, calmly and smoothly. Relax your solar plexus . . . abdominal organs . . . lower back . . . hips. . . . Relax your legs and feet. . . . Now relax your whole body. Relax and be aware.

(1 minute)

Imagine you are surrounded by positivity, boundless well-being, and light. Now bring your attention to the space above your head. In that space, feel an infinite ocean of healing, love, and light.

(1 minute)

Feeling that presence of wholeness, light, well-being, and contentment, become aware of your body breathing.

(1 minute)

Remaining completely relaxed, the next time your body breathes in, feel a stream of this boundless presence of light and joy descend into the top of your head and slowly down your spine to the center of your chest. As you exhale, feel it fill your heart—your spiritual heart (in the center of your chest). Feel light, love, and positivity flood that space.

On your next inhale, feel all negativity, sadness, and suffering lift out of the heart center. Feel or see it move up the spine to the top of the head. As you exhale, release all of the darkness that's been sitting on the light of the heart, release it out into the universe. Without forcing the breath in any way, continue the practice. Do not control your breath. Just let it be effortless. Do not breathe fully or forcefully. Allow your breath to be silent.

On the inhale, absorb universal intelligence, healing, and light; on the exhale, feel it fill the heart.

On the next inhale, all the darkness that clouds the light of your heart floats upward to the top of the head, and as you exhale feel it disperse out of the body and mind.

(Please continue for 2 minutes)

If it's helpful, add the mental repetition of "I am." On each inhale, feel "I," and on each exhale, feel "am." The Sanskrit words for "I am" are *so hum*. You may find that either of these phrases helps you connect more deeply to the light in your heart. If you find the English or Sanskrit words distracting, don't use them.

(3 minutes)

Gradually notice your breath becoming softer and shallower. As your mind becomes quieter, gradually begin to feel or see yourself "entering" the practice. You are no longer in your head doing the practice, trying to imagine it; you are immersed in it. Your imagination and intention have slowly opened the door to the experience of a new and boundless world. More and more you feel connected to light and freed of the weight of old thoughts, hurt, and darkness. Continue to do the practice.

(3 minutes)

Eventually sense that the light in your heart is permanent. Feel that you *are* the light that is beyond all suffering. With your mind tranquil, you open to a new world. You see that while the external world, your mind, and your breath come and go, the light of your soul is eternal, unchanging. The less you try and the more you just allow it to be, the more you will enter into the light of your heart.

(1–3 minutes)

Sense that this light is a "light beyond all sorrow." When your mind has become still, rest in this light in your heart. At this point, stop doing the technique of moving awareness up and down the spine and simply rest in your heart. If you notice that your mind is still busy or that you still feel any darkness overshadowing the "light of the heart," continue the technique—effortlessly.

(2 minutes)

Relax. In the final stage of the meditation, feel complete contentment, so full of love you need nothing or no one to feel content.

Rest and feel the feeling of wholeness and complete joy.

(2 minutes)

When you are aware of yourself resting in a sense of wholeness and contentment, you are ready to access *dhi.*

TECHNIQUE FOR ACCESSING YOUR *DHI*

Step 1. Once your mind is quiet, just be there, rest in this state for a moment. Be effortless and completely aware. Sense your body at rest, your mind at ease. Now cultivate a feeling of delight; feel surrounded by and filled with love. Remember, though, that you are not *trying* to imagine a different or hopeful reality; you are simply being aware of the highest truth—unconditional love. At this time, sense you have no worries or concerns. Just feel the joy of being. Knowingness rises out of this bliss. Deep contentment, love, and wholeness precipitate wisdom. Before you go to the next step, feel complete.

Step 2. From a feeling of complete wholeness and ease, sense the presence of intuition, the voice of conscience, or your inner teacher. Often, this presence is experienced as an inner light or a flame. Whether or not you see a flame, from the deep calm of meditation sense that a timeless part of you has the perfect answer to any and all questions. For the next moment or two, feel this flame or presence dissolve all doubt, insecurity, or fear. Just rest in the presence of your inner teacher and sense it subsume all distraction. Sense this "knowing presence" become more concentrated; see or feel it located somewhere in your body. It might be in your gut, in your heart, or perhaps somewhere else in your body. Rest there and feel, see, or hear the quiet confidence of knowingness.

Step 3. Abiding in this authentic inner wisdom, assume that you know, and need to know, nothing. With openness and compassion, unburden yourself of expectations and the need for a particular outcome. Expect nothing; be open to everything.

Step 4. While abiding in that presence, silently ask your question with clarity and precision. Be aware of your mental tone of voice. Assume you are posing the question to someone (or something) that has infallible insight and that this someone or something is your dearest, wisest, and most caring ally. Ask with confidence, trusting that it wants nothing more than the best for you.

Step 5. Remaining completely relaxed, hold your awareness in your "wisdom center" and listen for an immediate response. If you felt a response but you weren't able to hear it clearly or grasp it, center yourself and ask again. If after two or three times you still don't have an answer, return to Step 1, where you rest in the quiet of the ease you achieved through meditation, and start again.

Step 6. Once you have received a clear and definitive response, slowly come back. Acknowledge that you've been somewhere special, done something important. Take a moment to recognize and

thank your inner guide. Honor your voice of wisdom. Like all
things in life, whatever you appreciate grows. If you did get more
than one answer, write them all down and then circle the one that
you sense is the most authentic.

That's it. That's the process. Don't obsess about what you heard or
didn't hear. Simply ask yourself, "Can whatever was revealed to me be of
help, and if so, how?" I recommend writing both the question and the
answer down right away so that you can look at them later. If you heard
more than one answer, it is important to learn to separate rational
thoughts from responses that are intuitive. Your inner guidance speaks to
you from a more subtle, more all-encompassing place than your intellect.
As I mentioned earlier, its answers very often come to you as a flash,
whether through something you hear, see, or feel. Write down all of your
responses, even if they contradict each other, and consult them in the
days that come. The more often you look back on your answers and see
that your inner voice was right, the more your trust in it will grow, as will
your skill in perceiving it.

I strongly recommend that you access your inner voice whenever you
are unclear, facing a decision, or embarking on anything significant.

Here are some additional thoughts on accessing your *dhi:*

- After doing this exercise a few times you'll know the location
  of your wisdom center; you'll be able to connect to it immediately.
- Pose your questions there, as if you were opening a sealed en-
  velope that contains the answer and guidance from a higher
  source.
- Keep in mind that your inner voice has to be nurtured. If you
  have neglected to listen to it for a long time, it may be harder
  to hear. This is similar to what happens to a child who has
  been repeatedly ignored; he or she will simply shut down in
  response. Only when the child begins to feel acknowledged
  will he or she gradually begin to share with you.
- Use meditation to access your *dhi* regularly, even if you don't
  have a specific question to ask. If you do this, you'll find that
  your inner wisdom will guide you in your life in helpful and
  often surprising ways. When you don't have a specific ques-

tion, just meditate to still your mind and ask if your inner guidance has anything to tell you. Then be open to its response.

For intuition to grow as a force in your life, you have to learn to honor it. One form of neglect is not taking the time to hear it; the other is ignoring what it is telling you to do. This means that for your inner voice to become an increasingly powerful presence, you have to act on its vision. This is the pivotal point of the next chapter: the power to know what to do is only valuable if you also exercise the power to do what you know.

CHAPTER 18

THE POWER TO *DO* WHAT YOU KNOW

Roxanne and I would speak about once a year. It was pretty much the same conversation every time, which if you were to boil down my side of it could be summed up in a single word: "When?" Roxanne wanted to start a new chapter in her life; she even knew what she wanted it to look like. It was the same vision year after year. Yet she kept finding reasons not to act on what her heart was telling her to do. That's why in each conversation I found myself asking her, "When are you going to do it, Roxanne?"

Roxanne's dream was to move away from the East Coast city where she lived, the job that had long ago stopped satisfying her, and the life that was even less fulfilling. Roxanne said she wanted my guidance, which is why she asked to speak to me every year. Yet despite the fact that she had formulated a Dharma Code ("I make a difference in the world"), had a very clear *sankalpa* ("I have a fulfilling and creative life that nurtures and inspires me. I love where I live, I love what I do"), and felt at least some sense of an inner voice guiding her, she insisted on holding on to the idea that she didn't know or couldn't be sure that moving was in her best interest.

Year after year in our conversations she would explicitly and implicitly communicate the pain of maintaining the status quo while also brimming with excitement and wonder at the possibility of starting her life afresh in a place where she could "see the ocean." It was almost like hearing two different people who never bothered to listen to each other. One was somber and practically hopeless about her life conditions; the other was almost childlike in her enthusiasm about what it might lead to if she were spontaneous and followed her heart. If Roxanne could really have heard herself, it would have been obvious that she had little to lose and everything to gain by moving forward. Yet for more than four years she did not.

Each time we spoke I reminded Roxanne of the methodology of learning to listen to her heart. More than once I walked her through the exercise of learning to listen to *dhi* that I described in the previous chapter, and before each of our conversations was over I did all I could to encourage her to trust what she heard in her heart by acting on it.

In Roxanne's defense, responding to her inner guidance did require courage. Starting a new chapter in her life would mean leaving a secure and well-paying job, a few close friends, and a city she knew well to move to an unfamiliar place with no job and no friends.

Roxanne would often acknowledge her fear about making such a move. However, time and time again, she would say that it wasn't her fear that was stopping her; her justification for not moving was that she didn't feel as though she had the clarity to know whether or not it was actually her conscience talking.

After three years of the same justification for not pursuing her dreams, I felt it was time to be blunt. "Roxanne, your conscience does not want you to be unhappy indefinitely. I understand that you want to be absolutely certain that it is your conscience that is speaking and telling you to move. Meanwhile by not listening to it, you've been able to stay 'secure' with a steady job in a city with which you are familiar but in which for years you've been unhappy. After sitting quietly and listening to your heart, you've heard, 'Move on, seek a change'—the prospect of which elates you. What makes you think it isn't your heart?" I then told her, "For three years you've *known* what you've wanted to do. You've heard your heart speak. However, you have consistently chosen to confuse your fear of acting with *not* knowing.

"Roxanne, you do know. But you're afraid, and I understand that, and it's okay. It's perfectly legitimate to be afraid. But your heart has spoken. You're just trying to avoid doing what it's telling you. Until you act

> . . . .
>
> *The actual bridge that spans the gap between you and the fulfillment of your desires is the actions you take, informed by your inner guidance and wisdom.*
>
> . . . .

on it, you shouldn't expect to be happy. No one who indefinitely ignores his or her heart should. When all is said and done, our only responsibility is to our inner guide or teacher, and to respond to it by doing what it is telling us."

That conversation was the turning point. Roxanne finally listened to her heart and not her head. While fearful of starting a new life without the safety net of a specific job or place to live, she did it anyway. Four months later, Roxanne e-mailed me that she was going to move. Not long thereafter, she wrote me a second e-mail from her new home on the West Coast.

Dear Rod,

Doors have opened without much effort and I feel supported as I've never felt before. So many blessings . . . I had an interview for a job at [a major west coast university]. I got the job! Work starts January 12, which means I have a whole month to explore the area, study, read, and enjoy myself!

Then there's the beauty of the land: hills and water, water and hills all around. No matter what happens, I can just climb up a hill, stare at the water, take it all in, and be in tune with the universe. The feeling all along is that I haven't come this far alone, and whatever happens—good, bad or indifferent—is all good, and I'm not alone. I'm still not used to feeling this way, but it's a great feeling.

Roxanne, much to her amazement, transitioned gloriously to a new life. Yet it nearly didn't happen, and none of it could have happened until she took action. That is the central message of her story. It serves as a potent reminder to anyone wanting to fulfill a goal or, in a larger sense, to live a truly satisfying and meaningful life: no amount of aspiration toward a particular goal can bring it to fruition without some action. This is the very definition of spirituality in action: to put into action what you *know*, what you are certain of at the core of your being. If you fail to respond quickly enough to inner guidance, you may lose the specific opportunity to which it was trying to lead you. It doesn't really matter whether you're writing a novel, trying to raise money for a worthwhile cause, starting a spiritual practice, or mending a broken relationship— the best and most effective time to act is when you first hear the call to do so. This is when the forces of Nature are most powerfully aligned to help you achieve your aim.

When all is said and done, the steps of *The Four Desires* are a preparation, a foundation for your fulfilling your intentions; they set up the conditions to achieve your desire. The actual bridge that spans the gap between you and the fulfillment of your desires is the *actions* you take, informed by your inner guidance and wisdom.

Julie's Story

Julie had begun to feel as though she would not find a way to get "unstuck." Her children were now at an age where they needed her less. Her career as a restaurant and food critic for a newspaper had come to an abrupt end due to a change in management. She felt anchorless, as she put it, "drifting toward an all too familiar shore of depression." Yoga had become a partial refuge, but whatever solace it provided her would go by the wayside the moment she tried to meditate. Mostly it was one frustrating experience after the next every time she tried. In class, she couldn't help comparing herself to everyone else in class who "seemed to get it." She would sit there, her mind "buzzing and swooping," interrupted only by her imagining the sublime experiences that the person next to her was having.

Julie's world for the past three years felt like it had been getting darker by the month. That was when she heard about the Yoga of Fulfillment workshop. Julie's vulnerability at the time made her utterly teachable. This meant that despite having little or no evidence that the elements in the process could or would be of much help, she carried on and completed every step that I've led you through until now.

Relax into Greatness was her breakthrough along with her *sankalpa* ("My writing is reaching more people than ever with new information that will inspire and teach"). The following are her words:

The first thirty minutes of Relax into Greatness were sheer torture. My head throbbed, my throat itched, I wanted to cough or vomit, but no one else was moving. I dared not shatter the silence by running to the bathroom. At one point you [Rod] had us count back-ward from fifty, telling us to start over if we got lost. I never got be-yond forty-one. Another meditation failure. But, hey, when it came to meditation, I'd made friends with failure.

Then during a later part of the practice, where you walked us through another series of steps, I can't recall them but I do remember you saying something like, "Just quietly be aware; relax and watch. Something may unfold." I then dropped into the deepest silence I had ever felt. It felt good. Suddenly a long dark tunnel stretched out before me. I couldn't believe what I was seeing, but somehow I had become so relaxed that I felt able to trust what I was seeing, where I was being led.

At the end of a tunnel I saw a light and the vague outline of a woman. I couldn't see her face or body through the darkness, but in-tuitively knew she was beckoning, calmly encouraging me to come to her. I lost touch with time, with my body, with my customary frus-tration surrounding meditation. I do not know how long I watched the woman. I felt she knew me, everything about me. A surge of recognition passed through me: That woman was me! It was as though I was seeing a future version of myself, a dim outline but clearly recognizable. A wave of ease overtook me.

A part of me was struck by how much my future self was unlike my present self. I sensed that I was or, more to the point, *could* be a powerful, welcoming woman of infinite love, compassion, and for-giveness. I felt in that moment that a part of me was encouraging me to walk forward and ignore the circular detours of fear that had plagued me so much of my life, and never more than in the past few years.

I later realized the full significance of what I had experienced. My vision of my future, loving self had shown me that I did have the courage to set aside my fears and begin a new, bolder way of living. I could now trust myself. There was a way to move forward, and it would lead me to new and wonderful worlds. The gift of that day has not stopped reverberating even after eight years. I see the woman who guided me that day often now.

I've moved beyond my work as a restaurant critic to become an award-winning cookbook author with three books under my belt, successfully launched two children into adulthood, and served as chairman of the board of a local nonprofit. I'm currently starting a new business, and I'm excited about the prospects for success.

In the years since, thanks to practice and more work with you, I've developed a regular meditation practice, and continue to engage in continued self-inquiry. *Stuck* is no longer a part of my vocabulary. With every year I feel a deepening sense of purpose.

Julie's story of a vision revealing a more enlightened, free, and courageous version of herself that was prepared to lead her to a far more productive and fulfilling life may be inspiring, but it should not distract you from the critical point about what it actually takes to achieve most worthwhile desires. It's about action. Had Julie not taken action by responding to what she had seen or heard within, the message she had received from her conscience would have led to little other than a vague and mysterious memory.

Again, the message is that once you have seeded your unconscious with an intention, it will provide you with clues and opportunities, which must be responded to by taking action in a timely manner. Julie's accomplishments of the past years have had everything to do with her decision to act upon her inner guidance.

> . . . .
>
> *The best and most effective time to act is when you first hear the call to do so. This is when the forces of Nature are most powerfully aligned to help you achieve your aim.*
>
> . . . .

In order to understand how we ordinarily make our choices, let's look at the yoga tradition's powerful insights into the three distinct ways human beings decide.

Stages of How You Decide

The faculty of the mind that makes decisions, in the Vedic tradition, is called *buddhi*. The term comes from the root *dhi*. As we've seen, *dhi* means "knowingness"; it also means "intelligence." *Buddhi* refers to the part of the mind that "decides"; it is not the reactive or instinctive part (the part that causes you to duck if something is about to hit you in the head, for example). Unlike the reactive part of the mind, *buddhi* deliberates, if only for an instant, before making a decision. It does so by drawing upon what it normally uses to orient itself, namely, past experiences and self-perception.

Buddhi has three stages of development. Each stage is defined by the criterion it uses to make decisions. The first stage is defined by instant gratification. At this stage, after accessing all its options, *buddhi* will decide how to proceed based on how best to avoid things that are unpleasant and, as much as possible, to experience things that are pleasant. It will base its perception of pleasant and unpleasant on its identification with past experiences and by doing all it can to maintain its sense of self, no matter how limited or misinformed its perceptions may be.

This is exactly what drove Kristin, time and time again, to decide to stay in her marriage. An abusive childhood and a father who later abandoned her left her with an acute sense of low self-esteem as well as the impression that she should accept a family unit that was fractured. As unfulfilling and destructive as this impression was, it was all she knew, and because of its familiarity, it provided her with the most comfort.

At that stage of its development, Kristin's decision-making faculty or *buddhi* had been unable to overcome the limitations of her upbringing and self-image to help her make better choices. Thus Kristin kept making the decision to stay even as the situation got worse and worse.

Kristin's self-destructive method of choosing is not all that unusual. It is the basest of the three criteria for making decisions, the kind of thinking that has sparked many wars, the formation of inner-city gangs, drug use, child abuse, infidelity, and any other example where a choice to do or not do something is based on trying to defend or assert a false or limited understanding of one's self or one's relationship to the "other." Making choices in this manner is a failure of clear perception as much as it is a failure to exercise self-discipline, or at least a failure to delay gratification for a greater good. Practically everyone is born with their *buddhi* at this stage of development; some of us learn to outgrow it.

At the next stage of development, *buddhi* operates from a greater level of self-control and what could be called maturity. At this level, it is capable of considering a larger picture of the world within which it must operate. Thus it is now oriented toward making choices that are most beneficial or helpful to us in the long run. Stepping out of its preoccupation with the pleasant and the present, it bases its decisions on what will support our personal, social, and spiritual growth. To a much greater degree, it understands the limits of selfish and self-centered action.

At least for some, parenthood compels us toward this kind of think-ing, as it eventually did for Kristin. When parents place love for their children above all else, it often allows them to transcend even the neglect (or worse) that their own parents may have visited on them.

At this second level of development, *buddhi* is rooted in a more evolved philosophy. One example of this might be, "Do unto others as you would have them do unto you." At this stage, because decisions are based on a larger sphere of awareness, they can take shape around family, organization, society, and so on. We make sacrifices, shifting away from the pursuit of immediate gratification above all else and accept that there will be times when delayed gratification will better serve us and our pur-suit for more happiness. Ultimately however, self-interest is still the *bud-dhi's* main agenda at this stage.

The final stage of development of *buddhi* is demonstrated in the lives of Mahatma Gandhi, St. Francis of Assisi, and Socrates as well as in the life of anyone who has embodied the noblest characteristics of hu-mankind. Their decisions—their words, actions, even their thoughts—transcend the personal and are motivated purely from an unerring commitment to the highest truth or conscience. The commitment to embody virtue above all else, to be a living expression of the highest truth, no matter the consequences, is the hallmark of the highest level of *buddhi* as decision maker. At this level, choice and an approach to life are not determined by the hope of making one's life easier or more pleas-ant in either the short term or the long run. Socrates, when presented with the option either to stop questioning the citizens of Athens to bring out the highest truth or to be put to death, did not hesitate. He chose death.

By completely embodying the highest and most evolved stage of *buddhi,* and therefore by serving conscience above all else, Socrates and others whose lives embody the highest truths are the most exceptional of human beings. Few ever embody this level completely, but on those oc-casions when we do allow our conscience to be the arbiter of our actions, we become a vehicle for *dharma*—the intelligence that pervades and sus-tains all things—in which we create a lasting legacy that is the fulfillment of our ultimate purpose (our own *dharma*).

This is what Julie was, in some measure, able to do when she no longer let fear and doubt shape her choices. By standing courageously and lovingly for the self that she envisioned she could be, she ventured into what for her was an uncharted world, and she was rewarded in countless ways.

Acting, based on the voice of one's conscience, is the central message of the Bhagavad Gita. The text makes it clear that doing so defines the path that we must follow to fulfill our destiny. It will not always be easy, but there is no other way if you are committed to finding and living your life's highest purpose. The value of living a life inspired solely by conscience is unsurpassed. Why don't more of us act this way? One reason is because a part of almost all of us resists change. In the next chapter, we'll look at why—and how to overcome our resistance to it.

CHAPTER 19

. . . .

THE COURAGE TO CHANGE

The physical practice of yoga is said to include some 840,000 postures, ranging from the simplest you can imagine to postures so extreme even the most advanced gymnast might find them out of reach. Every body is different, so no matter how flexible or strong you might be, some postures will be easier and more accessible for you than others. But after working with tens of thousands of individuals, I can tell you that the single hardest yoga practice is the same for everyone. It's called *change.*

I've taught millionaires who in material terms could accomplish in a single day what many of us would be thrilled to do in a year, yet when it came to fulfilling their wish to work less so they could spend more time with their families, these immensely powerful individuals become practically powerless. I've worked with meditators who could sit for hours and access profound physical and mental stillness yet were unhappy and terribly frustrated with their lives, far from being at ease when it came to building a meaningful, inspired creative life, a career, or financial security. Making a million dollars is not a big deal if you are a multimillionaire, yet learning to relax, find peace, and settle into your heart can be. On the other hand, stilling your mind is not a great accomplishment if you've been doing it for years, but learning to engage fully in the world in a way that is enriching and truly fulfilling may be difficult for you. This is why the journey of becoming a more complete and capable per-

son may be the greatest challenge that any of us can ever face. It is also
the most rewarding.

Have you practiced Relax into Greatness yet? Have you done any of
the meditations? If you have, congratulations. It is an accomplishment to
do something new, especially without
someone there to motivate you and without a roomful of other participants doing
it with you. It requires a powerful willingness to act in your own best interests.

> . . . .
> *The single hardest yoga
> practice is the same for
> everyone. It's called* change.
> . . . .

If you have yet to do Relax into Greatness or any of the meditation practices, it
confirms my point about the challenge of
change. You may have been impressed by the case I made for them, and
you may have made plans to do them, but for one reason or another you
have yet to actually do them. I haven't given up hope that you can and
will. Knowing how powerful and beneficial these techniques are and how
good you would feel if you were to do them, I pray that you will do it.
And that you will do them soon.

The point is that it is challenging to create and maintain a new trajectory, especially during the period prior to experiencing the fruits of
your new endeavor. In the interim, it takes courage. Courage is almost always a necessary ingredient of change. Fulfilling your potential and
achieving your destiny demand that at some point you stand on your
own and become your own leader. No one other than you has ever had
precisely the same *dharma*. Thus, while you may find others with whom
to share your life and your love, ultimately true growth requires you to
clear your own path. Your blossoming will need to be unlike anyone
else's; just as every double helix of DNA is unique, so is every person's
path. Even identical twins have their own, individual expression.

There is a relevant teaching on this concept in the *Hatha Yoga
Pradipika,* the seminal book of the Hatha yoga tradition. The text describes six impediments to success in yoga. The first four that we need to
overcome are straightforward:

- Overeating
- Overexertion
- Talkativeness
- Unsteadiness

There is nothing particularly surprising about the list so far. Avoiding these obstacles leads you to a more balanced life. But the final two impediments might surprise you. They speak directly to the need for each of us to discover and live our uniqueness. The last two things to avoid are:

- The company of common people
- Adhering to rules

Avoiding the "company of common people" is not a prescription for being a snob. Nor does it mean that you cloister yourself away from the world. It is based on the truth that everyone is uncommon—if they are willing to be. The only common people are those who have not yet found the courage to live as their uncommon selves—the very courage that Julie's conscience was beckoning her to act on and which she ultimately embraced.

A fundamental intent of this teaching is to remind us that we need to guard against losing precious time, and equally precious energy, by trying to be someone less (or other) than who we are supposed to be. If you are not mindful, the "company of common people" can distract you from your mighty purpose, the creative urge within you to fully express your unique self. Conversely, the company of extraordinary people reminds you of the power of having faith in your own uniqueness and acting courageously from it.

Similarly, refusing to adhere to rules doesn't mean that you will become a lawbreaker, dangerous, or violent. Indeed, if you are listening to your conscience, which is by definition an expression of *dharma*, wisdom, and compassion, it could never guide you to do such things. Not adhering to rules means guarding against only those "shoulds" that will lead you to anything less than your best life. It means learning to be a singular force, committed to living your soul's urge to be and become. There may be nothing as empowering and quite so liberating as exercising this capacity.

The following exercise will help you see the power of living this way. It will give you an experience of what it's like to act on your inner guidance, an experience that for many people leads to following this practice in their daily lives. Unlike the other exercises I've given you, this one requires that you be sufficiently prepared before you start it. Specifically, in order to do the exercise you first need to be confident that you are able to hear your conscience or inner guidance. This means that you've used the method I gave you in Chapter Seventeen to access your *dhi*, you've noted the results, and you've seen how often the inner guidance you've received has been trustworthy. If you are to a point where it is consistently trustworthy, you can be confident that when you feel you're hearing your inner voice—your conscience or intuition—you actually are; it's not your reactive mind, your rational mind with its collection of "shoulds," or even your imbalances talking.

You may be ready to do the following exercise now, or you may need to keep using the method from Chapter Seventeen to access your *dhi* until you know that you can trust what you are hearing. But regardless of where you are in the process of building confidence in your *dhi*, please read this exercise now.

EXERCISE: FORTY-EIGHT HOURS OF FEARLESS ACTION

The directions for this exercise are very simple: now or sometime in the near future when you're ready, dedicate forty-eight hours to constantly responding to your inner voice. This means saying yes to those things your inner voice says yes to, and no to those things your inner voice says no to. It is not your job to question your inner voice; it is your job, for those forty-eight hours, not to deny what you hear. If it says turn off the television, you turn off the television. If it says take a walk, you take a walk. If it says to be kinder and more patient with your wife or husband, do it.

> *The only common people are those who have not yet found the courage to live as their uncommon selves.*

As long as you are listening to your conscience, you do not have to worry about it leading you through a course of action that will be in opposition to your best interests or to the greater good.

Remember, you are not responding to what you *think* you should be doing. You are not acting based on impulses conveyed to you from your rational or reactive mind, feelings, or emotions. Your intention in this exercise is to experience a sense of freedom in which your only allegiance is to the voice of your conscience, which is limitlessly wise and compassionate.

Again, please wait to do this exercise until you are confident that you are able to hear your inner voice. You need to be able to hear inner guidance without doing the meditation, because for the period of the exercise you are going to need to hear it continuously throughout your day, moment to moment. I also suggest not doing the exercise if you are in the midst of any serious life issues or under significant duress. In other words, before giving yourself permission to act on all your impulses, it's important that you feel balanced both physically and mentally, you have a degree of peace and serenity, and you are physically healthy and sleeping well; only then should you attempt this exercise.

If after forty-eight hours you find that you don't want to stop, you can extend it for as long as you like. Very likely you'll find it catapulting you to an entirely new way of being—freer, more powerful, more often in the right place at the right time.

Once the forty-eight hours have come to an end, I recommend writing in a journal about your experience. The following questions may help you reflect on it and get a clearer idea about your relationship to "knowing what to do" and "doing what you know."

- In what ways were the last forty-eight hours different?
- How completely did you listen?
- How well did you respond to inner guidance?
- How often did you listen to it and how often did you not?
- Where were the particular areas of your life where you felt stuck or less responsive to your inner guidance?
- What did you learn from the exercise?
- What did it tell you about the way you live or the way you would like to live?

John's Story

John came to the Yoga of Fulfillment to, as he put it, "break out of his old life." Interesting, since he himself was a life coach. He was busy all the time, scheduling clients from morning till night, in large part because he needed the income. He had an expensive car, a nice home, designer clothes, and a habit of spending money freely. He shared with me that he believed he lived this way to reward himself for working at something that had become unfulfilling, and to create the appearance for his clients of being a model of success. John's whole life had become defined by what he did; he was always "on." He hadn't had a meaningful relationship in several years.

By the time I met him, John was running on empty, and had been for longer than he cared to admit. "I was burned out," he told me. "I'd run out of ideas about how to revive my career, something I used to love but that had become little more than an obligation that provided an income."

According to John, the moment his life turned around was when he did the forty-eight-hour exercise:

> The exercise was a godsend. It crystallized all the work of the process and gave me permission to act fearlessly. Trusting that a part of me other than my intellect had the answers and would guide me to the solutions I was seeking lifted a giant burden off my shoulders. It opened a door that gave me a vision of an entirely new way of thinking and being.
>
> Over the past decades, I was endlessly preoccupied with trying to know what I or what others should and shouldn't be doing. I had completely suppressed all play and spontaneity in my life. I had become an incredibly lonely and judgmental person.
>
> The exercise changed me forever and propelled me toward an amazing life that I didn't even know to look for. When I started the exercise, I had a Dharma Code: "I brighten the light of this world, I bring love, laughter, and discovery to everything I do"—a stretch from what my life was at the time. I also had a *sankalpa:* "I love what I do, and I do what I love"—also a stretch. Before having any sense of what I would do or even that I would change careers, I made the vow to listen to my inner voice. It wasn't hard once I finally chose to do it; it was a relief.
>
> After two days of doing the exercise I realized how inept I was— how few times I actually did what you were asking us to do. The listening part was not that big a deal; my conscience has always been a strong voice. But after one complete day I realized exactly how little I responded to it. I decided to keep going, if for no other reason than to experience one complete day of not hesitating to act based on what I heard.
>
> I decided to extend the exercise for a week, vowing that I wouldn't judge, resist, fight, ignore, or avoid where I was being led. Although I didn't do that week perfectly, it didn't matter. I felt so good and filled with so much possibility that I decided not to stop.

One of those days I sat down and spent a few hours writing a story for Max, my sister's six-year-old son, that I planned to read to him. I was surprised by how much I enjoyed it, but didn't give it much more thought. I decided to extend the exercise for another week.

The decision to honor the part of myself that I had long discarded almost instantly was bringing something in me back to life. Immediately I experienced a flood of inspiration. All week long I started feeling a rush of ideas for more stories. I normally would have not paid attention to the inspiration, but I listened and jotted down my ideas whenever they came to me. I wanted nothing more than going back to the quiet of writing. Even when I would be on the phone with clients, my mind kept wandering back to what other stories I could come up with for Max.

I heard that I needed to buy a journal, so I did; to spend more time in Nature, so I started hiking a ton. I heard that I should stop paying attention to the news and reading psychological journals when I was away from work. I started playing volleyball, cooking, throwing weekly dinner parties.

At some point I stopped doing the exercise consciously, but not before the die had been cast. The dinner parties introduced me to a whole set of new friends, one of whom heard I was writing in my spare time and said that a dear friend of hers was a brilliant illustrator and that the two of us should meet and possibly collaborate.

Before I met Maureen I was enjoying one of the most productive and exciting phases of my life. Because I was already feeling so happy when we met, I felt comfortable around her. I had not stopped life coaching, but I knew it would become more and more part time as I explored other areas professionally. Maureen and I fell in love. A year later, we finished our first book together and have since published another. I now do life coaching part-time. The strange thing is that now I love it again, but when I tell people what I do, I never say I'm a life coach. I either tell them my Dharma Code—"I brighten the light of this world, I bring love, laughter, and discovery to everything I do," or I just say, "I write children's books."

My work, my family, and all the blessings in my life today are rooted in that month or so of walking past my fears and taking action.

REFLECTIONS ON TRIANGLE POSE

. . . .

Trikonasana

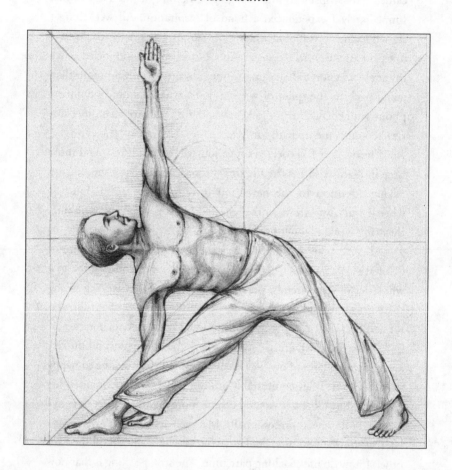

Triangle Pose is one of the foundational postures of *asana* practice. It is commonly used early on to help students understand and experience the dynamic forces behind a rewarding yoga practice. For students of all levels, Triangle Pose creates an immediate awareness that yoga is a profoundly tactile experience—one that not just reaches your hamstrings, in this case, but energizes the whole body and mind. As simple as the pose may appear on the outside, once you're in it you discover internally the

power of dynamic tension. This is the principle of action and counterac-
tion, which you learn in the pose by experiencing resistance versus freedom, stability versus expansion, and grounding versus aspiration—the
opposing forces that each of us has to find a way of bringing into balance
in our lives in order to truly thrive.

The central physical intent that these opposing actions are directed
toward in Triangle Pose is the lengthening and expansion of the spine.
Approaching Triangle Pose with this in mind, you discover that for every
intention there is at least some resistance to that intention. Triangle Pose
typically reveals tension or resistance in the following areas: the hamstring of the front leg, both sides of the waist, the core of the body, and
the ribs, chest, neck, shoulders, and upper spine. In each case, the tensions or patterns we hold in these areas are the result of postural imbalances, mental and emotional stress, gravity, aging, and the subtle
influence of inertia, which to some degree affects all of us at one time or
another.

The discovery of these or any other limitations in the posture serves
to awaken us to the fact that the very thing that is challenging us or holding us back can be our catalyst for growth to become something greater
than we have been. Learning to challenge your resistance in the posture
lights the same inner fire that allows you to overcome your limitations
and to fulfill your potential in life.

The *Yoga Sutras,* the seminal text of the yoga tradition, tell us that the
more intensity you direct toward attaining the goal of yoga, the more resistance you overcome, the faster you will achieve your desired ends. Similarly, whatever your goal, whether it be Triangle Pose, any other pose, or
life itself, the more intensity you generate toward achieving it, the more
you increase the likelihood of attaining it. However, I should point out
that one of the things that the practice of *asana* teaches us is that applying greater intensity does not always mean working harder. In fact, increasing the intensity of our *relaxation* is a vital part of achieving any
goal, be it mastery of a particular pose or something in life you truly aspire to achieve.

Triangle Pose is a beautiful embodiment of the universal principle of
intention overcoming the resistance to it.

PART V

. . . .

FREEDOM

FROM FEAR

. . . .

CHAPTER 20

MAN PROPOSES, THE UNIVERSE DISPOSES

A little more than a decade ago, in what seems like a different life, I was living in Los Angeles, had never been married, and had no children. I was as busy as any yoga teacher in the country, impassioned about what I did, and in many ways fulfilled. Nonetheless, I found myself thinking about the future and wanting clarity about it, so one day I decided to create a picture of exactly what I wanted life to look like ten years down the road.

Using a pen and a sheet of paper, I made a quick, rough sketch of an ideal future. I believed that drawing would be the best way to give voice to my intuition, to let it, rather than my intellect, paint the details of an ideal future home and work life. Before starting to sketch my dream life, I wasn't attached to any particular concepts about what it would need to be. All I knew was that I longed for a productive and purposeful life, a life that served the greater good and at the same time was richly rewarding both spiritually and materially. I cleared my thoughts, opening myself to inner guidance, and put pen to paper as fast as I could. Less than ten minutes later, I had a rough sketch of a ranch-style home surrounded by open space, overlooking snow-covered mountains. My wife-to-be and I were standing on a deck, watching two small boys playing. Nearby was a corral with a few grazing horses. The drawing also included sketches of a variety of yoga DVDs, meditation and Relax into Greatness CDs, and a published book.

The sketch excited and surprised me. My intuition had revealed some things I'd already known I dearly wanted and others that I'd never really thought about. The yoga DVDs and meditation CDs were no surprise, and I'd always known I wanted to be a father and happily married. On the other hand, I was unaware of wanting to live in the country or write a book. Nonetheless, it did feel as though inner guidance had provided me with a vision of a future that, if I could fulfill it, would give me the kind of life that was right for me.

I resolved that someday, perhaps in ten years, I would manifest all the elements in my drawing. However, everything about my circumstances at the time—living and having a career based in Los Angeles, as well as being single—was a very real reminder of just how far away my dream was from reality.

The dream seemed such a distant fantasy and ten years seemed so far away that I put the sketch and the dream aside. I made the decision to focus on doing what was in front of me instead of staring and fixating on the drawing of a future that I might or might not ever have. I shelved the drawing and within a month lost track of it completely. I had had an inspired depiction of the future, but the demands of my present life were all-consuming.

In the years that followed, my teaching grew exponentially, and so did the amount of traveling I did. During that period, I opened a yoga studio in Los Angeles, a rather counterintuitive choice for someone wanting to leave Los Angeles. During that time, I also had two serious romances, both of which ended unceremoniously. As my obligations, responsibilities, and teaching schedule grew, I would occasionally remember the drawing and wonder whether or not my present circumstances were moving me closer to the dream it depicted. It certainly didn't feel that way; if anything, my success as a teacher and the time I spent on the road seemed to be moving me away from my vision of having a family and living in the country, not toward it.

A lot was about to change.

Four years after making my sketch, I got married. Two years later, I was blessed with the birth of twin boys, Jaden and Theo. Yet as wonderful as their coming into the world was—the realization of at least a part of my cherished dream—it also marked a time when it became clear that my marriage was failing. By the time the boys were fourteen months old, I made one of the most difficult decisions of my life and filed for divorce. Thus began the most turbulent and challenging of times. I spent the next year working through a long and difficult divorce, which led to my becoming a single father with full custody of Jaden and Theo.

While moving the three of us into our new home, I came across the sketch I had done six years before. I stared at it and pondered all that had happened. The life in the sketch seemed no less idyllic, but more remote than ever. However, I had little time to dwell on what might have been or what was still to come. Too much demanded my attention. I was starting life over and was responsible for two young lives.

My first priority was to provide my sons with a new beginning as well, to create a loving home for them. If I wasn't teaching, I was cooking, diapering, bathing, shopping for groceries, reading bedtime stories, or doing one of countless other chores related to raising two healthy, precocious boys. Anyone who has been a parent, let alone a single parent to twins, can probably sum up the experience in a few words. Two that come to mind are *exquisite* and *exhausting*—very exhausting. Life consisted of little other than teaching, parenting, and lack of sleep.

During this period, when the rest of my life was exclusively about giving to my sons and to countless students, my daily practice of yoga and meditation became my sole opportunity to nurture myself. I did it even if it meant getting up at 3:00 a.m. to practice while the boys were asleep. Meditation in particular was my manna. There were two other key sources of nurturing without which I'm not sure I would have survived. My mother, who filled in far beyond the duties of grandma, was one; the other was doing the processes that I've shared with you in this book. Being able to refer to and receive guidance from a clear and defined life purpose during what was the most challenging time of my life helped me stay the course. My Dharma Code, "The fire of Spirit is invincible. It lights my way and empowers me to brighten the light of others. Teaching, creativity, leadership, laughter, and love are how I serve humanity and God," was my rudder in very rough and uncharted seas. It was the one thing that kept me going in the direction of my higher purpose even while meeting the day-to-day challenges of a life that was taking everything I had.

I must have been doing something right, because about eighteen months later, deep in the throes of being a single dad, a friend introduced me to her best friend—a woman who unexpectedly turned out to be the most extraordinary person I am quite certain I will ever know. A little more than a year later, Gina and I would marry.

The next year, Gina and I tried on two separate occasions to buy a home in Los Angeles. In both instances, our offers, despite being above the seller's asking price, were turned down. We started to wonder if it wasn't a sign to leave Los Angeles.

We began an extensive search for the right place to settle and raise our two boys. Ultimately we decided on the Pacific Northwest. A month before we planned to return for a second trip to Seattle to buy a home, a conversation with a friend reminded me of my love for Colorado. It inspired me to take Gina, Jaden, and Theo for one more reconnaissance mission, if for no other reason than to make sure our decision to live in Seattle was the right one.

The moment we touched down in Colorado we felt at home. We found natural beauty, a great environment in which to raise and educate the boys, a progressive community, a home we both fell in love with, and—last but certainly not least for someone who had spent nearly four decades in Los Angeles—no traffic. As I write this, for nearly four years we've been living in the home we fell in love with.

Recently, while walking to my office, I suddenly remembered the sketch I'd made twelve years ago. I literally stopped in my tracks. Recalling each of the details of the picture I had once made of my dream future, I realized it was a nearly exact depiction of the life I was living—the only exceptions being that the horses I see are not my own but my neighbors', and the book you are now reading had been written but not yet published.

That day, I realized that I had fulfilled my dream, and that, amazingly, it had taken almost exactly ten years from the day I'd drawn the picture, just as I'd said to myself it would. With the benefit of hindsight, I recognized something I pointed out in the part on *sankalpa*: once I articulated my dream and committed to it, I set about responding to inner guidance as consistently as possible, and the universe set into play an endless series of events that brought my intention to fruition. And throughout the decade it seemed to me that each circumstance—every single one, including the worst of the trials and tribulations—had needed to occur before my intention could come into being.

There is another lesson in this story, though—a plain and stark reality: fulfilling your dream is often less than easy, and the road to it can be, at the very least, circuitous. In the interim between my "proposal" and its "disposal," life took many twists and turns, and I encountered major challenges, few of which, while I was going through them, appeared to be leading me toward the future I longed for. Before I met Gina—more than six years after making my sketch—there wasn't the slightest hint that I was even on the way to being happily married, much less that my family and I would one day be thriving in the mountains of western Colorado.

I lived what is an essential lesson for anyone staking claim to an intention who then finds himself or herself living in the gap between desire and fulfillment. There are no guarantees how quickly or easily you will get what you want, or even if you will get it. The truth is that some dreams never come to fruition and some turn out to be hollow after they are fulfilled. The dreams that are achieved often take more time for us to achieve than we would like, and sometimes, in the process of materializing our desires, they require us to give more of ourselves than we knew we had.

The Bhagavad Gita, like the Old and New Testaments, teaches us that no matter how pure your intentions, it is impossible to live without having to confront challenges, confusion, difficulty, and even tragedy. We all discover at an early age that we don't always get what we want, let alone when we want it. There is no ancient wisdom, modern technology, personal power, or income bracket that will absolutely ensure that we will always attain what we want, or if we do attain it, that we will be able to keep it.

> . . . .
> *If you are to have fulfillment and, perhaps more important, if you are to sustain it even while living in a world that is not wholly dedicated to your happiness and security, you will have to develop a way to approach life skillfully.*
> . . . .

The president of the United States, His Holiness the Dalai Lama, and Bill Gates are not above being affected by forces beyond their control, and neither are you. There will always be someone or something to answer to; whether it is a group, a political party, Nature, or even God Herself, something holds at least some of the cards that determine your fate.

You can never be completely insulated from the sudden shifts of life: a downturn in the stock market, a natural disaster, a terrorist attack, the unwanted end of a relationship, a sudden and severe illness, or the death of a loved one. This is why *The Four Desires*, a book about fulfillment and getting what you want, must also explore how best to cope with life's disappointments. If you are to have fulfillment and, perhaps more important, if you are to sustain it even while living in a world that is not wholly dedicated to your happiness and security, you will have to develop a way to approach life skillfully. The yoga tradition provides powerful methods and strategies to help you do so.

"Yoga is the breaking of contact with pain," says the Gita. This means that there is a way to experience freedom and sustain fulfillment even while dealing with life's inevitable complexities. Thus we now turn our attention to what happens when our desires meet the world's unpredictability, because the simple truth is that our desires (more specifically, our relationship to them) are the cause of most of our suffering. The relationship between desire and suffering is a seminal part of Vedic, tantric, and yogic traditions. Learning how to apply these teachings to our own lives is as much a yoga practice as doing any postures or breathing techniques.

"How do I find lasting happiness in a world that doesn't always provide what I want?" "Is there comfort to be found in an unpredictable world, and if so, where?" "How do I remain positive and live joyously while I wait for my dreams to be fulfilled?" "How do I avoid letting disappointment weaken my resolve?" "Where should I turn when things appear hopeless?" Throughout the ages, spiritual and religious traditions have provided a single answer to the questions posed above. In Western terms, it is called surrendering or letting go. The Sanskrit term for this is *vairagya,* which can also be defined as "dispassion, detachment, or nonattachment." (Throughout this part I will use these words interchangeably.) As the Gita tells us: "Seek refuge in the attitude of detachment and you will amass the wealth of spiritual awareness. . . . There is no cause for worry."

Pause for a moment. It would be easy to pass over the words "no cause for worry" and not fully appreciate their significance. Instead, let the meaning of the words sink in. Try to imagine worry and stress no longer being part of your life. For most of us, this would mean an entirely different life from the one we are living. The idea of living worry-free is fantastic! For most of us, it's also a theoretical proposition; most of us are not capable of being dispassionate 24/7. However, to the degree that we can

. . . .

"Yoga is the breaking of contact with pain," says the Gita.

. . . .

learn to apply dispassion, non-attachment, and surrender to our daily lives, it is a prescription for worry-free living, one that can affect everything from the most practical and worldly aspects of your life to the most spiritual. The Gita paints a clear depiction of its reach and impact when someone is able to master it.

> The awakened sages call a person wise when all his undertakings are free from the anxiety about results; all his selfish desires have been consumed in the fire of knowledge. The wise, ever satisfied, have abandoned all external supports. Their security is unaffected by the results of their action; even while acting, they really do nothing at all.

This teaching on *vairagya* is so extraordinarily rich and touches so many key principles that improve the quality of your life that I will be drawing from it to weave the theme of non-attachment through the chapters in this part of the book. Most important, I will use it as a basis to provide you with accessible tools to make non-attachment a stronger presence in your life. Despite how often you may have heard terms such as *letting go, surrendering,* or *non-attachment* in the past, the whole notion of what they mean may still seem a bit abstract; if you've tried to apply them, you may have found yourself unable to or perhaps even resistant to the very idea. If you don't yet know exactly how non-attachment can contribute to your having more of the life you want, this part will make non-attachment clear and teach you how to apply it.

THE *VAIRAGYA* EXERCISE, PART I

Before we move on to the next chapter I'm going to ask you to do Part I of a simple and extraordinarily effective two-step exercise. The exercise requires a pen and a sheet of paper. The first step will take you less than fifteen minutes to complete. It will be the basis for Part II of the exercise in Chapter Twenty-one. When you've completed the second part, you will have a clear experience of what *vairagya*, non-attachment, is in practical terms and how you can apply it.

Recall an experience in your past that had a significant negative impact on you. It can be any experience, circumstance, or condition that was emotionally, physically, or spiritually hurtful or debilitating. Write one paragraph detailing the particular experience or event, then write another paragraph describing its aftermath, detailing ways it has inhibited you or had a harmful or less than constructive impact on your life.

You may choose to write about a childhood experience, perhaps your parents' divorce, financial stress in your family, or the death of a close family member. You can also write about something more contemporary, such as a disappointment at work or with your family or a strained financial situation—anything the aftermath of which has caused you to feel, think, or act in ways that either sabotaged you or kept you from recognizing who you truly are and could be. The experience you write about doesn't need to be your life's most dramatic or intense. You can write about such an experience if you want, but again, you don't have to. Whatever experience you choose, you will probably have feelings about it. You do not have to choose one that feels emotionally overwhelming or that automatically carries you to a very dark emotional place.

Remember, write only two paragraphs: in the first, you'll describe what happened; in the second, you'll describe how it negatively affected you, your relationships, your view of the world, your self-esteem, or any other area of your life.

Once you've written the two paragraphs, save them and put them aside. You've completed Part I of the exercise.

CHAPTER 21

YOUR MIRACLE ANGLE

Stage One of Non-Attachment

Non-attachment is said to be one of the essential characteristics of the Divine. Imagine embodying absolute non-attachment. Imagine, at any instant, being able to release all hurt, fear, and anything else that might inhibit you from residing in complete freedom and the fullness of your spiritual glory. Consider what life would be like without even the tiniest fragment of doubt standing in the way of living boldly and confidently. What if you no longer looked to the world or to anyone in it for validation? What if you felt you had nothing to prove, nothing to hide, no one to hide from?

If you were capable of this experience, you would be the highest embodiment of *vairagya*. But it's not necessary to embody non-attachment in the absolute sense for it to help you in your life.

Indeed, I think about non-attachment in terms of stages, like the stages of a rocket launching from earth. Scientists talk about a rocket's launch as stage one, stage two, and stage three of liftoff, with each stage the rocket rising farther and farther away from the earth and its gravitational pull. Similarly, as you apply *vairagya* in your life, you are drawing away, in successive stages, from the pull of all the things that have kept you from living life to the fullest.

At stage one *vairagya*, non-attachment releases the weight of disappointment and emotional pain. At stage two, it becomes a catalyst for emotional growth and prepares you to achieve the things you would otherwise not be capable of achieving. Stage three is its ultimate expression. This is where it becomes a foundation for connecting to the ultimate Reality. At this stage, non-attachment becomes the means by which you fulfill *moksha,* the fourth and final desire, the longing for true freedom. Each successive stage of non-attachment helps you navigate both the calm and turbulent seas of life with more and more fulfillment.

A Famous Example

Steve Jobs, co-founder of Apple Inc. and former CEO of Pixar Animation Studios, delivered the 2005 commencement address at Stanford University. The theme of *vairagya* is woven throughout his account of his personal journey. With great candor, he described how devastated he felt after getting fired in 1984 from the company he co-founded and the terrible feeling of failure that resulted. To make matters worse, his firing was highly publicized; the toll of the embarrassment was so great that it even led him to seriously consider leaving Silicon Valley. However, with time to reflect, Jobs realized that he still had a passion for his work, and he made the decision to begin all over again. Eventually, he came to recognize that being forced to leave Apple was actually a gift; relieved of the burden of his past triumphs, he turned his attention to beginning anew, which led to a phase of unbridled creativity. What followed was a series of groundbreaking innovations, and to Jobs starting two new companies: Pixar (which pioneered computer animation) and NeXT (which was eventually bought by Apple and would provide much of the core technology for many of Apple's most popular products today).

Steve Jobs's success—his ability to chart a path to an entirely different and rewarding future—is a very clear illustration of this stage of non-attachment. His ability to "let go" of both the devastation of failure and the weight of his previous accomplishments was, as he emphasized, the key to creating the opportunity that awaited him. It was what allowed him to find the right perspective from which to view all that had happened. Before he could do that, however, he had to experience hardship and let go of everything that had defined him up to that point.

As the months passed and his view of the events cleared, Jobs was able to release what the earlier quote from the Gita calls the *"anxiety about results.*" As a consequence, he was able to see the good in his situation. Not long after, the burdens of failure were supplanted by a feeling of excitement about starting over again, no longer bound by the known. He felt free.

By not holding on to his feelings of embarrassment and loss, Steve Jobs propelled himself into an extraordinary life course. The rest, including Apple's phenomenal success, is history. Being dispassionate, which the dictionary defines as "not influenced by strong emotion, and so able to be rational and impartial," allowed him to turn the page on what *was* and move on to what *could be*—an altogether new and rewarding chapter in his life.

The Physiology of Non-Attachment

What do anger, depression, apathy, pessimism, loneliness, anxiety, despair, insomnia, tension, colitis, addiction, susceptibility to infection, an array of skin disorders, heart disease, headaches, backaches, weight gain, and loss of sex drive all have in common? They are all relieved the more we practice non-attachment. Research has even found that non-attachment is a common psychological characteristic in people who live to be one hundred years old or more. Yes, people who make non-attachment a regular part of their lives live longer—and, dare I say, more happily!

Can the right perspective, illumined by the fire of *vairagya*, really make the difference, helping you rise out of the ashes of failure and setting the stage for fulfillment, as it did for Steve Jobs? The answer is yes. The following stories further illustrate why and how non-attachment or surrender is so extraordinarily helpful.

Alan, the son of my teacher Mani, is a masterful teacher in his own right. Many years ago, he was asked by one of his students to try to help a grieving friend of hers, Martha. Not long after Alan arrived at her home, Martha began describing the emotional pain and suffering she had been enduring since her husband's death. "Since he died," she told Alan, "I've been so distraught and overwhelmed that I've been barely able to leave my apartment. I'm afraid to go out of the house, or ashamed, or perhaps I just don't have the strength to face the world anymore. I don't know if yoga or you can help, because I'm not even sure if I want help. To be honest, I believe I've lost the will to live. Since losing my husband, I really can't find any reason to be happy again. I live in the shadows of his death. I can't imagine that ever changing."

Martha kept talking this way for more than thirty minutes. Before she was done, Alan began feeling the weight of her hopelessness. A bit shaken, he finally asked, "How long ago did your husband die?"

"My husband? He died thirty years ago," she responded. Her words were a jolt back to reality. Thirty years?

Martha had been carrying the loss of her husband for more than three decades. She had found no reason to spend the rest of her life without the burden of losing him because she could not let go of the sense of who she had been with him. If he was gone, so was she—all because she had not let go.

Compare her story to that of the mother of Divya, a student of mine. Divya's mother is one of the most energetic, lively women I've ever met. The truth is, I have never called Divya's mother by her first name. Like many people who spend even a little time with her, I call her Mom, for the simple reason that she so completely embodies the best and most joyful characteristics of a caring mother. (She also happens to be from India, where it is not uncommon to call someone with a powerful maternal presence Mom.) In her eighties, Mom has as big a love of life as anyone you can imagine. Her laughter and the sheer pleasure she exudes are infectious. She has a large circle of close friends, exercises regularly, is an amazing cook and hostess, dances, attends temple on a regular basis, and loves just about everything she does.

> *Every perspective on "reality" (good, bad, or indifferent) is just that, one perspective—one degree of what is actually 360 degrees of reality.*

Only on the rarest occasion have I heard her speak about being a widow. When she does talk about the man to whom she was married, it is clear that she was no less in love with him than Martha was with her husband. The two of them, Mom and Martha, represent two very different ways of looking at similar situations. The difference has everything to do with the angle from which they are choosing to see their lives. The two very different choices led to two very different lives, one brimming with love and joy and energy, the other filled only with the emptiness of loss.

THE *VAIRAGYA* EXERCISE, PART II

You are now ready to do the second step of the exercise you started in the last chapter. For this part of the exercise, you will need a pen or pencil and one or two sheets of paper.

I'd like you to write again about the same experience or event you described in the first exercise, but this time I'd like you to write one or two paragraphs about how that experience has helped you—or about how it *could* help you, could contribute something to your life. In other words, you will look at it from a perspective opposite to the one you took in Part I of the exercise, when you wrote about its negative impact. Doing this may require you to dig deep. If the circumstance you chose to write about earlier was particularly tragic or extreme, it may be a struggle to find anything at all redemptive about it. Perhaps its only positive impact is that it taught you that you could survive, and that your life can be a living testament to others that they too can survive tragedy. If that's the case, then write about that.

It's essential not to start writing until you have found a perspective and a way of relating to the experience or event that is authentic to you. I suggest taking as long as you need to gain insight into how you can view it as contributing something constructive to your life. Once you have an understanding of the potentially positive effects of the incident, start writing. It's not necessary to describe the circumstance again; you've already done that. Instead, write only about how it was or could be helpful, how it empowered or could empower you.

Here are some questions to ask yourself to help you decide what to write.

What has the experience or event taught you?
How has it strengthened you?
How has it helped you in your relationships with other people?
How has it helped you spiritually?
Has it helped you to become more compassionate, more ethical, more inspired, more capable?
Has it helped you not to take yourself or every setback in life too seriously?

This exercise can be easy or quite challenging, depending on the circumstance about which you've chosen to write and whether or not you've been able to come to terms with it. If you've dwelt on the pain associated with the event without ever having achieved any resolution about it, finding a way to look at it from a viewpoint that focuses on its potentially positive effects may take a while. Give yourself whatever time is required to find that new perspective before you start writing.

After you have written one or two paragraphs from this new perspective, please ask yourself the following questions. (There's no need to write down the answers.) Were you able to find at least one positive way to view your circumstances? Was it hard to find? Until now, have you ever chosen to look at your experience from a positive perspective? If not, why not? Have you consciously chosen not to or has it been an unconscious decision? Would it help you to start viewing it from this new perspective from this point forward? Is there anything to gain by not looking at it from a positive, healing, or proactive perspective?

When you've answered these questions for yourself, you've completed the exercise—and you've experienced firsthand what it's like to apply the first stage of non-attachment.

Pain, disappointment, and even anger are very human responses to some of life's circumstances. But to the extent that we are able to engage in stage one non-attachment—as exemplified by Mom, by Steve Jobs, and by what you have written about the positives that you can see when you look at your experience from a new viewpoint—we become what the Bhagavad Gita describes as "wise, ever satisfied," and more capable of having our "security . . . unaffected."

It is an abiding principle of *dharma* that *every* experience can help you grow and move you closer to who you are meant to become. The key to being able to do so is being willing to surrender, to be dispassionate, to let go of your attachments to the past and your expectations of the future. In doing so, you find a point of view, as you did in the exercise, that will help you live more freely and fully. I call this positive point of view the Miracle Angle because it allows us to see the potential for something good in even the most painful experience.

Everyone who has ever overcome hardship or adversity has done so in large part because he or she has chosen, consciously or unconsciously, to live from a Miracle Angle. This is what Steve Jobs did, but it's only fair to point out that what he had to overcome at that time pales in comparison to some of the tragedies and challenges that countless human beings have had to confront.

Loss of loved ones, war, prejudice, abuse, disease, and poverty are just some of the hardships that life presents. Yet for some extraordinary human beings, even extreme circumstances such as these did not prevent them from living inspiring, sometimes glorious lives—lives that illuminate the world in ways that often benefit all of us. The writings and lives of Anne Frank, Viktor Frankl, and Nelson Mandela, for example, remind us that we are capable of living from the best in ourselves in even the most dire situations.

Finding a Miracle Angle requires you to not be bound to any single perspective. In part this means accepting the idea that it is practically impossible to know and ever fully understand why a particular event happens. I once heard someone say, "If man could think like God, man would be God." As much as we may try, it is all but impossible for mortal beings to ever completely know why we have to live through what we have to live through. Only an enlightened mind escapes the confines of limited perception. Stage one non-attachment provides a glimpse of this aspect of enlightenment by freeing us from holding on to a particular interpretation of a situation.

Even death is open to interpretation. Many people assume there is only a single way to view death—as a sad loss, an event to mourn, dark, somber, funereal. However, in some parts of the world, death is celebrated—viewed not as a loss but as life's most sacred and auspicious time for spiritual awakening. In much of India and Tibet, for example, death is seen as an opportunity, a precious doorway that, if walked through consciously and with the support of prayer and sublime awareness, becomes an opportunity for spiritual salvation. And there are also cultures that respond to death with dancing and drinking. Close friends and family get together to laugh, cry, and have a party.

If even death has no single meaning—if there is no one particular angle from which it should be seen—then it's clear that there is no right or wrong way to interpret any experience; there is only what is helpful and what is not. Every perspective on "reality" (good, bad, or indifferent) is just that, one perspective—one degree of what is actually 360 degrees of reality.

This explains why there is more than one way to respond to widowhood. The two women whose stories I told responded in different ways because one had found a Miracle Angle and one had not.

How do you find your Miracle Angle? It's not complicated, and you've already done it at least once. In Part II of the exercise, when I asked you to find a positive perspective on a painful situation that at one time you interpreted as negative, you were finding your Miracle Angle. The more often you choose to live your life from the Miracle Angle perspective, the more happiness, ease, and opportunity you will experience.

The easiest way to gauge whether you are seeing things from a Miracle Angle or what we could call your Grievance Angle is whether or not you're suffering. If you are suffering or if you have become stuck in a nonconstructive point of view, it means that either you have not found your Miracle Angle or you have not fully embraced it. If it is the former—if you are struggling to find a perspective that lifts your spirits and empowers you—you need to look harder. It is there. Remember, every situation has at least one Miracle Angle. If, on the other hand, you have found what you think is a Miracle Angle yet you feel that you are still not at peace with your situation, it means you are not yet living from it. Once you detach yourself from your grievances, however justified they might be, and you abide within the perspective of your Miracle Angle, you will find yourself embracing the gift of life and living it more fully.

Both of these steps require *vairagya* or non-attachment. Not only does non-attachment help lift some of the weight of your suffering, it also links you to the curative force of free will. When you're attached to a single point of view, you're also attached to a single way of responding. You assume that there's only one course of action—or inaction. When you let go of that particular point of view or those feelings about what you've experienced, you open yourself to a new perspective from which you are empowered to choose a new way to respond. In other words, you become aware that you have free will, that you can find a Miracle Angle and choose to act from it.

The following story is another example of how choosing to live from your Miracle Angle can make all the difference.

Jennifer's Story

When she did Part I of the exercise, Jennifer chose to write about the breakup of her marriage and the difficulties she was now having at work with Howard, her ex-husband. After years of struggling as a couple, they had agreed to end their marriage amicably and find a way to work together at the art gallery they had started years earlier. Ideally, they both would have liked for Howard to buy out Jennifer's half of the gallery, but he couldn't afford to, so they decided that he would pay her a salary and apply it toward the purchase price until the day he could do the buyout. Although running the gallery had previously been the one area in which they had been reasonably compatible, not long after they started their new arrangement Jennifer began to feel as manipulated at work as she had felt in their marriage. As time went on and Howard moved into a new relationship and she did not, Jennifer's experience of working with him only got worse. But her own financial situation made it all but impossible for her to leave the gallery.

The following is an excerpt from Part I of Jennifer's *vairagya* exercise, the description of her challenging circumstance from a negative perspective, her Grievance Angle. Jennifer had a lot of practice being negative about her life, and the exercise gave her a chance to get it all out:

When Howard and I ended our marriage, I saw it as a clear sign that I would never be happy and thrive in a relationship. For the nearly ten years we were together I had done all that I could: I was patient, giving, affectionate, I worked on myself, and did everything for the relationship; it was never enough.

Not long after our divorce, Howard found another woman, and they've been together now for over three years. They seem happy. Knowing that he's with somebody else makes me feel inadequate, like there's something wrong with me and that I am incapable of having a healthy relationship. The end of our marriage takes me into the dark feelings of loss that I've had most of my life. Beginning with the death of my father when I was four, I've always had a feeling that I wouldn't be taken care of and that things would not turn out all right. Being single again and, even worse, having to depend on him to treat me fairly and for my income bring out the worst feelings I have about myself. It becomes harder and harder to take care of myself and to do the things I need to do to stay healthy and have a positive outlook in life. I've stopped reaching out to people, especially to the people that do love me. I feel boxed in . . . it feels like there's nowhere to go and little hope.

The following is from Part II of Jennifer's exercise when she wrote about the divorce from her Miracle Angle. Be prepared: these two versions read like they were written by two different people. They weren't.

The fact that I'm no longer together with Howard is a sign that I am healthy. I chose to end it. If anything, that is a sign that I've grown and that I'm unwilling to stay in a destructive relationship. It also means that at least some part of me believes that I can take care of and fulfill my own needs. I don't need a man or someone to save me. This is the first time in my life where I took action that shows I believe it. Not being with Howard signals a new chapter in my life.

Seeing him at work every day and depending upon him to write my paychecks is not evidence of being a victim or being incapable of having a loving relationship. I chose to make this arrangement because it pays my bills and I get to work at the gallery I co-founded in a field that I love. It is proof that I've grown and am capable of fulfilling my own needs and that I have finally accepted myself as the savior I've always been looking for. I choose to see the challenges of working with him as small compared to the pain of the past when I had so little faith in myself.

Every day is a reminder that all things now are possible that never were. The best of my life is ahead of me.

Two years later I ran into Jennifer and she told me how much of a difference having a Miracle Angle had made in her life. Not long after she had adopted a new perspective, her ex-husband had begun treating her differently. They still work together, but now their relationship is working and she has grown in ways outside the relationship—professionally and emotionally—that are truly fulfilling her. She's had several relationships in the meantime, and although they've not been lasting ones, they've been a magnificent break from her past because in each relationship she has felt nurtured.

Jennifer's Miracle Angle allowed her to change her perspective on a situation that had been debilitating her. By giving her permission to see it differently, her Miracle Angle illuminated for her all that was good about herself and her life. Once she affirmed that she was on the right path, she then became more capable of fulfilling her dreams of being self-sufficient and nurtured.

Getting to this first stage of *vairagya* is as easy—and as hard—as making the decision that you will find your Miracle Angle and then committing to live from it.

"Reshape yourself through the power of your will," the Bhagavad Gita tells us; "never let yourself be degraded by self-will. The will is the only friend of the Self, and the will is the only enemy of the Self." Why is the will both friend and enemy? Because, as we've seen, it can lead you to make either positive or negative choices about how you will respond to life—*and the choices you make about how you will respond determine everything.*

I strongly urge you to find your Miracle Angle as often as possible. Don't sleep on your resentments, pain, and suffering. Before going to bed each night, clear your mind and find the Miracle Angle from which to look at any circumstance that is troubling you. You might not instantly feel uplifted by the change in perspective, but it will provide you with the understanding and acceptance from which you can move forward with a clearer sense of purpose.

CHAPTER 22

FULFILLMENT MAY BE WAITING FOR YOU (TO CHANGE)

Stage Two of Non-Attachment

It is a day I'll never forget: being in a long, sterile hallway of the Los Angeles Superior Court building, in the midst of my divorce proceedings. Our judge had asked us—myself, my attorney, my soon-to-be-ex-wife, and her attorney—to mutually decide on several logistical matters concerning our court case. Sitting alone on a bench as our lawyers faced off, I noticed that the hallway was filled with other attorneys and their clients going through the same strained ritual.

If you've never been in or near divorce court, it's probably hard to imagine the level of rage exhibited by divorcing couples just outside the courtroom doors. Inside, in front of the judge, everyone is on his and her best behavior, but outside the anger and disgust are palpable and often audible. It's not uncommon to hear couples, who perhaps only months ago were choosing the menu and flowers for their wedding, angrily voicing their disgust about their former spouse for all to hear.

There, amid all these soon-to-be-divorced combatants and their attorneys, I recall thinking that I would never under any circumstances put myself in a position of having to return to this scene again. There was no doubt in my mind. I would never marry again. Yet . . . I have married again, and it is a glorious marriage at that. Why?

As absurd as the idea of ever getting married again seemed to me at the time, there was also the matter of the sketch that I had drawn of my future. A part of me—deep inside, beneath the pain and sadness of a failed marriage—still wanted to know and share in the love of a family, and to live with my family in a place near snow-covered mountains. I had not thought about that dream for a while; nonetheless, the seeds of my resolve had been planted. Sooner or later, there would be only one thing left to change before I could have what I wanted—me. I would need to change. Nothing played a bigger part in helping me do that than surrender.

Nature is always teaching us who we are meant to be. In reality, although it may always be teaching us, we are not always receptive to learning. To be teachable, we need to be as open to learning from failure and pain as from success.

> . . . .
>
> *If you resist learning your lessons in their gentler forms, life is more than prepared to teach you through ever-increasing hardship.*
>
> . . . .

Life's lessons come in many forms. If you resist learning your lessons in their gentler forms, life is more than prepared to teach you through ever-increasing hardship. If nothing else, Nature seems to know that hardship will eventually break down your resistance and loosen your attachments so that you finally embrace the lessons that life has long been trying to teach you. It is only when you apply non-attachment that you become truly teachable. At that point, you are able to change not only when it becomes excruciating not to, but also when subtle signals of love and kindness tell you that change will be beneficial. Even the tender voice and needs of a child can become your teacher, as I was to discover.

Like Steve Jobs, I had a choice about how to respond to my circumstances. The experiences of my first marriage could have embittered me and prevented me from marrying again, or made me a less fit husband the second time around. Many people get married more than once, but often they bring their pain, mistrust, and anger along with them. Fortunately, I kept practicing what my teachers had taught me about how to stay open to life's directives. Meditation and taking time to reflect on what I had done right as well as what I had done wrong in my first marriage were part of the process. I chose to keep learning.

There have been plenty of teachers in my life. There were my principal teachers, Kavi Yogiraj Mani Finger, Yogiraj Alan Finger, and Pandit Rajmani Tigunait, with whom I formally studied as a student, and the thousands of students I've taught, who have served as my teachers as well. Life experiences have also been teachers: my first marriage, a painful divorce, and—above all others—my sons, Jaden and Theo. Raising my two boys as a single father and seeing to it that their needs were met could not have been a more powerful teaching. *Vairagya* helped me realize that if I was going to have what my heart truly wanted, I needed to become a different person.

If I was going to accept and learn from the painful lessons of my first marriage, I had little choice but to change. I had to grow. I had to want different things, especially what I looked for in the person with whom I could be content sharing the rest of my life. My sons prepared me to see and then embrace Gina and all her remarkable qualities, which only a few years earlier I might have missed. Without the lessons Jaden and Theo provided, I would have certainly missed fulfilling the dream laid out in my sketch. They helped me see that nothing was more glamorous and attractive in a woman than the qualities that would make her a true partner, one who could completely love and nurture the boys and me, and who was fully capable of appreciating the love we felt for her.

Jaden and Theo were my lighthouse. Their needs were a beacon, helping me navigate through dark nights and perilous waters to the safe harbor of the woman who was meant to be their mother and my future wife. By the time Gina and I met, I had become the person I needed to be to have what my heart truly wanted.

On the surface, the lesson of my story is that once you have an intention you must surrender your attachment to how it will unfold. Relax and know that larger forces are at play. Non-attachment rooted in a willingness to let go of even your most precious ideas and beliefs is the key element of stage two of *vairagya*. However, it's important not to confuse non-attachment with inaction or passivity. You have to *choose* to respond to what life offers you in the way of challenges. And sometimes nothing can be more challenging than the necessity of letting go of certain parts of your dream and accepting the fact that it may not be achievable in the form that you have imagined it—or even of letting go of certain parts of yourself.

Returning to the words of Charles Du Bos that I quoted earlier, "The important thing is this: to be able, at any moment, to sacrifice what we are for what we could become." The path to what we could become is often missed or not taken because of our attachment to who we have been until that moment.

Countless times over the years, I've worked with men and women who say, for example, that they want a relationship. They were even willing to work for it. Yet in spite of many disappointments they failed to see that they kept looking for the same person over and over again, which made it all but impossible for them to have what they wanted. This underscores how important it is to be willing to learn about yourself from your experiences and to grow based on what you learn. Being attached to a false picture of the kind of person they needed to be with, or to the part of themselves that needed to be disappointed time and again, these men and women did not have the freedom to find the kind of person who would actually fulfill them.

> . . . .
>
> *It's important not to confuse non-attachment with inaction or passivity.*
>
> . . . .

Stage two of non-attachment does not require that you relinquish your dream just because it may not have happened yet. It only means that you must stay open to learning about yourself while becoming a fuller and more complete version of you. This is why I said that stage two *vairagya* spurs emotional growth and prepares you to achieve the things you would otherwise not be capable of achieving.

How to Increase Vairagya

The breadth of ease and inspiration that *vairagya* offers us can touch any or all of our worlds: the external, our body, relationships and circumstances; the internal, our mind and breath; as well as the spiritual, our connection to Spirit, Universal Intelligence, or God. Different practices and actions affect one or more of these three worlds.

To enjoy more of *vairagya's* benefits in your relationships and other external circumstances, exercise the following: compromise, selfless service, charity, humility, compassion, and forgiveness (toward others and yourself).

To reap more of *vairagya's* benefits at the internal level, practice meditation, prayer, and relaxation. Relax into Greatness is an especially powerful technique. Do breathing practices that emphasize calm, smooth, and complete breaths. Do yoga, especially slower practices and restorative practices. Massage and self-reflection are helpful, too.

To enliven *vairagya* at the spiritual level, practice prayer, devotion (*bhakti* yoga, the practice of love and selflessness), and meditation. Of all the methods listed, the last two are the best and most direct at helping us reach the ultimate aim of *vairagya*, lasting peace.

CHAPTER 23

FREEDOM AND THE FIRE OF SELF-KNOWLEDGE

Stage Three of Non-Attachment

We are attached to our memories and to our resentments. We are attached to clothes we don't wear anymore, our work, our heartaches, our version of the facts, our habits, our anger, our fears, our political preferences, our disappointments. We are attached to the past and to our hopes for a better future; we are attached to our last argument with our spouse. We hold on to bad relationships and low-self esteem, and because of attachments we find it difficult, if not impossible, to stop doing certain things or being attracted to people who are not good for us.

It's hard to say when attachment begins, but it's clear that it follows us throughout our lives and very often grows in intensity. Take a cookie away from a two-year-old and you'll get a very visible—and angry—expression of attachment. As you get older, you generally become more discreet about how you express your attachments, but that doesn't mean they become any less powerful a force in your life. Just where does all this holding on come from? Why is letting go so hard?

Natasha's Story

I'd known Natasha for several years through a mutual friend. Although Natasha had never studied with me, one day she called to ask if I would be willing to help her mother, Sylvia. Sylvia was in her eighties, suffering from the advanced stages of leukemia. Three intensive rounds of chemotherapy and radiation had failed to slow the cancer's growth; at this point, her doctors were unwilling to give her any more treatments.

Natasha wasn't expecting me to cure her mother's cancer, just hoping that I could do something to help soothe Sylvia's emotional distress. Sylvia was living in her daughter's home and, Natasha informed me, was angrily mistreating everyone else who lived there, including Natasha's children. The psychological pain of Sylvia's terminal illness was taking a toll not only on Sylvia but on Natasha's entire family as well.

A few days after we spoke, Natasha led me into the room where Sylvia was bedridden. A silk scarf covered Sylvia's head. She was gaunt, her complexion gray, but I sensed a dignified elegance about her. She had the manner of someone who had lived a full and rich life. I also sensed Sylvia's embarrassment about her inability to do anything about me, a complete stranger, seeing her in her sleepwear. There was something else, too, something common to most of the terminally ill people with whom I have worked—a deep and subtle terror, just below the surface.

Natasha excused herself and left Sylvia and me alone, the social awkwardness between us heightened by Sylvia's physical pain and exhaustion as well as her unspoken dread. Neither of us could be certain what would come next. If only for a few seconds, time seemed to stand still.

It was hard for Sylvia to speak, but that didn't stop her from telling me right away that she had never meditated or done anything "spiritual" before, and she still wasn't sure why her daughter had asked me to see her. The truth was, we both knew I was there because she was dying.

> . . . .
>
> *Only when you begin to realize your fourth desire,* moksha *or spiritual fulfillment, are you able to see what lies beyond the world of impermanence, to touch upon the infinite.*
>
> . . . .

I was confident that meditation would help her, but I also understood that before she would do it, Sylvia needed to hear why. I began to describe, in a way that I thought she could relate to, some of what I've outlined in earlier chapters: a part of you is free, always at rest. It remains the same no matter what the condition of your body, your age, or your external circumstances; its nature is eternal. You gain access to it not through thinking, but rather through stilling the mind. Doing so allows you to access deep peace and to rest in the Eternal. Meditation is a systematic approach that allows you to still the mind and then unveil the deeper mysteries of life so that you can abide in lasting peace.

The more I spoke, the less Sylvia averted her eyes from mine. She began to ask questions and to smile, recounting her upbringing in the Greek Orthodox Church. Our conversation seemed to comfort her. Eventually I asked if I could lead her into meditation. She nodded.

I asked her to close her eyes. Closing my eyes as well, I began to talk her into meditation. Within moments, I could feel her mind and emotions settling. She was becoming more at ease. I led her deeper into the practice. A few minutes later, I opened my eyes and saw her resting in what was clearly a peaceful place. The expression of tranquility on her face reminded me that the thirst for peace is universal—something all of us, no matter our background, age, or station in life, deeply long for. I was touched by the fact that despite Sylvia's long and full life, she was experiencing something she had never experienced before. I knew that even the briefest glimpse of it could provide the one thing that at this time in her life she really needed: peace.

Twenty minutes later, the practice was over. Sylvia turned to look at me. There were tears in her eyes and, I could tell, a desire to express something that words could not convey. She smiled and quietly expressed thanks. Moments later Natasha, walking me to my car, wanted to know how her mother had responded. I told her that something positive had happened, but how and in what ways it would affect her mother I could not say for certain.

Two days later, Natasha called to tell me that since my visit Sylvia had been a different person, more at ease and in less physical pain. "The whole house feels different," she said. Sylvia wanted to know if I would come back. The next time I came, we recorded the practice through which I led her. I understand that she used it regularly for the next few months, until she passed—peacefully.

Addressing the subject of death, the *Yoga Sutras* teach, "Self-preservation or attachment to life is the subtlest cause of pain. It is found even in wise [i.e., enlightened] persons." Even if you are not consciously fearful of death, the yoga tradition tells us that attachment to life, the subtlest "cause of pain," overshadows every moment of our lives. This fear, which we are forced to confront directly when facing the end of our own life and when facing the death of others close to us, is also present in times of success and happiness.

Why fear death, something about which you have no experience or direct knowledge? The answer is, in part, that to the rational mind death is a void, the loss of everything you hold dear. When you die, there is no option to take your family or possessions with you, at least in the form to which you have grown accustomed. In short, death and the prospect of dying are the ultimate signs that you are finite and there is nothing you can do about it. Death is the great equalizer, a reminder that no matter what, ultimately none of us is in control.

Psychologists tell us that life's most stressful events include the death of a close family member, divorce, personal illness, and job loss—all examples of impermanence, of change foisted upon us involuntarily. Each, in its own way, epitomizes a lack of control—something your psyche, on a deep level, equates with death. It is for this reason, the *Sutras* tell us, that fear of death is the source of all other fears.

Fear of death is why, as human beings, we struggle with change— even those changes we are seeking to make. The end of our life is, of course, the most radical of all changes, and facing it is, if not the most difficult, certainly one of the most difficult challenges any of us will ever face. At such moments, everything hangs in the balance.

We are all part of an inexorable march through time. Spring becomes summer, summer turns to fall, and fall surrenders to winter. Sooner or later even the healthiest and most well-conditioned body wears out, the sharpest senses fade, the most learned mind must surrender to time. Life is finite, a precious gift, but inevitably an impermanent one. I consider it a profound privilege to help someone find peace as he or she struggles to accept this reality. The prospect of having to be mindful about our impermanence is not a very appealing one to most of us, however. If we are like Sylvia—and most of us are— we choose to more or less ignore the inevitability of death until, like an uninvited guest, it intrudes into our life.

> . . . .
> *This third and final stage of* vairagya *ennobles you with fearlessness and fills you with the freedom to follow your heart's call, knowing that a part of you is always safe.*
> . . . .

Fortunately, the ancient tradition teaches us how to face death fearlessly. The first step is to learn to see beyond death. Only then can you accept death and learn to live peacefully with it as an inescapable part of life. Through the ages, this very wisdom has been embodied by the Buddha, Jesus Christ, the Prophet

Muhammad, Mahatma Gandhi, and countless saints and sages, each of whom was able to approach his or her death differently than most of the rest of us will. What did they know that enabled them not to fear death as it approached? The answer, in the words of the Gita, is "the fire of knowledge"—the singular experience that dissolves all fear.

Achieving this, however, is not easy and goes against lifelong habits of mind. Even before you were able to say your own name, you began to believe in, and have an inherent sense of, who and what you are: you are your body, your thoughts, your emotions, your family, your job, your possessions—practically everything but your soul. This, in part, is why the first three desires involve your relationship to the material world. Only when you begin to realize your fourth desire, for spiritual fulfillment or *moksha*, are you able to see what lies beyond the world of impermanence, to touch upon the Infinite.

"Of the four aims, *moksha* . . . is the truly ultimate end, for the other three are ever haunted by the fear of Death," the *Vishnu Bhagavata* tells us. Sylvia's fear is the fear with which all of us live unless we fulfill the desire for *moksha*. The Vedas and most spiritual traditions point us toward the only source of peace, the Infinite, which is where we find our true Self. The soul is the door to the sacred, and it is the opening to *moksha*. The Gita tells us,

> The Self cannot be pierced by weapons or burned by fire; water cannot wet it, nor can the wind dry it. The Self cannot be pierced or burned, made wet or dry. It is everlasting and infinite, standing on the motionless foundations of eternity. The Self is unmanifested, beyond all thought, beyond all change. Knowing this, you should not grieve.

When death approaches, most of us recoil—but those who have tasted immortality within their own hearts do not recoil. Those who have this experience possess all the same physical and mental faculties with which you and I were born. The difference is that they have spent time stilling their search for temporary pleasure and found the bright fire of spirit.

It took twenty minutes for Sylvia to see that life was more than what she had previously known. That knowledge helped her more easily accept death and move beyond her pain and fear.

This third and final stage of *vairagya* ennobles you with fearlessness and fills you with the freedom to follow your heart's call, knowing that a part of you is always safe and "standing on the motionless foundation of eternity." Of all the practices that lead us to fearlessness, meditation and devotion are the most transformative in helping us to reach the highest stages of *vairagya*. Both methods, by dissolving the perception of separateness and freeing us from our attachment to the finite, ultimately reveal the deeper reality, where Essence, Spirit, Universal Intelligence, or God— call it what you will—shines brightly in all its light. Throughout the ages, devotees of various spiritual traditions have found it through unconditional love and a trustful surrender to divine Providence. Meditators have approached it through deepening stages of stillness, until one day they glimpse the Source of all.

Whether through surrender to a higher Being or through stillness, the pathway to *moksha* involves a letting go of "I" or "me" and all of its self-centered concerns, to experience a oneness with the Supreme. Once you are there, your heart and life are never the same. Throughout this book, I've shown you that one of the keys to fulfillment is experiencing that part of you that can only be known when your mind gets still. Meditation is the essential methodology to help you experience this. Here, I'll share with you an additional meditation technique, specifically to help you increase *vairagya*.

MEDITATION PRACTICE TO INCREASE *VAIRAGYA*

Come into a comfortable sitting position. If you are using a chair, be sure to have your lower back flush against the back of it so that your spine, neck, and head are in a straight line. Close your eyes.

Become aware of the space occupied by your body. Relax your whole body. Starting at the top of your head, relax facial muscles . . . neck . . . shoulders . . . chest . . . back . . . internal organs . . . hips . . . legs . . . feet. . . .

Now become aware of the space inside your body. For one minute do nothing but be aware of the inner space of your body.

(1 minute)

Once your body settles, become aware of your breath. Make sure you are breathing gently and smoothly and that there is no noise or unevenness in your breath. For a few moments watch the natural flow of the breath.

(1–2 minutes)

Once your mind settles on the breath . . . bring your attention to your abdomen. Allow your mind to rest behind your navel. Feel any and all thought, worry, concerns, distress, and distractions centered here—every thought and feeling that preoccupies your attention is concentrated in this space. Pause and feel the sum of your thoughts and feelings there for a moment or two.

(1 minute)

As you inhale, without forcing your breath, consciously let any anxieties, fears, anger, or thoughts—all the things you want to let go of—rise to your heart center. For a brief instant, pause your breath. See and feel violet light transform all your concerns into an awareness of complete ease and freedom; in other words, experience violet light dissolving all thought and worry; sense violet light invoking perfect clarity, inspiration, and wisdom. It is important to feel that the violet color—and the positive feelings you associate to it—is more powerful than, and is actively dissolving, the sum of your concerns.

Exhale effortlessly; see and feel the violet light rise upward and out the top of your head. Feel the letting go of all stress. Feel free of all pressures. Feel open and at peace.

Repeat the technique, remembering not to work or try. Simply do, without exerting any effort. Continue with the practice—effortlessly. At the end of each inhale gently pause and feel violet connect you to complete freedom and peace.

(1–2 minutes)

The more effortless you become, the more completely you will be absorbed in a growing sense of stillness and clarity, the more you will feel one with the violet light and the presence of freedom and lasting peace. With each cycle, feel yourself becoming more detached from all worries, fears, and doubts.

(5–10 minutes)

When you are aware that your mind has become completely quiet, rest in that feeling, surrounded by violet light. Eventually allow this light to lead you to a place where no limitations exist. Feel boundless and absorbed into the Infinite—a place of absolute peace and joy.

(1–2 minutes)

End of practice.

This meditation enables you to dissolve the bonds of attachment and open yourself to the Infinite, and thus become more free, more authentic, more spontaneous, and more willing to risk. In other words, by embodying more non-attachment, you become more fully yourself, and more able to respond to the call of your heart and intuition.

It takes courage to follow your heart and intuition and let them shape your life. Non-attachment summons this courage by moving you beyond *all* fears, including the fear of death. Freedom from the shackles of attachment and fear empowers you to take full advantage of the limited and precious time you have to create the life that your heart truly longs for. In the words of my teacher Pandit Rajmani Tigunait, "Only the fearless are truly alive."

REFLECTIONS ON HEAD-TO-KNEE POSE

. . . .

Janu Sirsasana

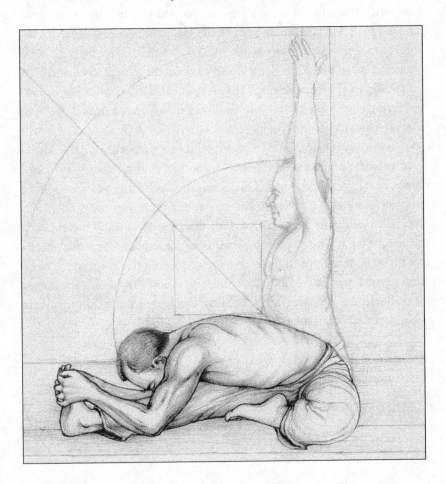

Head-to-Knee Pose is a powerful reminder that yoga doesn't need to be complicated or exhausting to offer you profound benefits. Like most forward-folding postures—and to varying degrees, all postures—*janu sirsasana* requires you to relax in order to fulfill your potential in it. In Head-to-Knee Pose, as in all other sitting postures, your body is in a very stable position. As a result, the action in the posture becomes more focused than it is in a standing or balancing posture, where your attention, and thus the work in the pose, is more dispersed. The primary focus of Head-to-Knee Pose is to lengthen and release contraction and tension held in the back of the straight leg, the inner thigh of the bent leg, hips, and most of the back, particularly the lower back. This may seem simple and straightforward; however, once you're in the pose you discover just how much muscular as well as physical tension you hold in these areas. The key to moving further in the posture is to relax, because once you become too aggressive or overwork the pose, you add to the resistance you're meant to overcome. By turning your attention to smooth and even breathing, with particular emphasis on your exhalations, your body gradually relaxes; tensions (both physical and mental) are released and you slowly move deeper into the pose.

As long as you continue to breathe smoothly, lengthening the particular muscles that the pose focuses on soothes your nervous system and stills even a distracted mind. Thus *janu sirsasana* brings you face-to-face with an invaluable life lesson: sometimes the more you relax, the closer you will be to your goal. Armed with this awareness, each breath, each moment you are in the posture, reinforces the sublime view that life affords you endless opportunities to let go. Applying this wisdom is a giant step toward greater freedom and possibility, one that allows you to see that sometimes the only things holding you back are the things you are holding on to.

PART VI

THE SECRET TO SUCCESS

CHAPTER 24

. . . .

THE ENDEAVOR TO BE "THERE"

Karen fulfilled her resolution. Recall that her *sankalpa* was "My family lives a life together that is abundant, peaceful, and simple, surrounded by a school community that shares our core values and is connected to the land." And that is exactly what she achieved. As you might recall, before she could fulfill her intention, Karen first had to resolve her inner conflict (her *vikalpa*) about it, specifically her desire to be a good daughter and her belief that she could only be a good daughter if she remained in the city where her mother lived.

I remember the day Karen came to a yoga workshop I was teaching and excitedly told me that she and her family had found and moved to the exact kind of community in which she had resolved to live. While telling me about having achieved the life change she had dreamed of, she was effusive, sharing with me the sequence of events that led up to it. Everything began, she told me, with a yoga workshop she had taken with me years earlier, in which I described a tantric view of how to measure the effectiveness of one's yoga practice. "You said there were three signs of an effective practice," she told me. "More joy, less fear, and a shortening of the time between creating an intention and having it come to fruition."

Karen said that weekend marked a turning point in her life. The most significant change for her had to do with inner guidance, which I'd emphasized in the workshop as being available to all of us, all the time, if we learn to cultivate our awareness of it. "I'd heard about inner guidance before," Karen told me, "and I don't know why this time it made such a difference. But I left the workshop sensing for the first time ever that I really did have an inner voice. It may not sound like much, but sensing that inner guidance and learning to listen to it were pivotal for everything good that has come since."

Karen's next step was to take the Yoga of Fulfillment.

The moment the course started everything seemed to click. My first epiphany came from the eulogy exercise. Writing from the point of view of a friend about all the things I hadn't accomplished, and why I hadn't accomplished them, suddenly everything became painfully clear. I'd spent most of my life basing practically every important decision in my life on other people's opinions and ideas. That discovery was my key to finding my Dharma Code, which five years later I still draw upon every day: "I receive Universal, loving guidance and channel it into the world with faith."

When Karen came to her first Yoga of Fulfillment workshop, she and her husband were renovating their house. Karen was anxious about it. Her *sankalpa* focused on what she wanted the renovation to provide: "I live in a beautiful, peaceful, renovated, and landscaped home that nurtures and supports our family on our true path." Looking back, Karen summarized: "The *sankalpa* worked better than I could have imagined. The house turned out beautifully. But it wasn't until two years later, when we sold the house, that I would see how it would wind up *supporting* us."

Two years after coming to her first Yoga of Fulfillment workshop, Karen attended a second one. That was when she uncovered her new *sankalpa,* her resolution to live a fulfilling life in the right community with the right educational environment for her family. Karen went on to describe to me the many links in the chain that led her to achieve this goal.

A few weeks after this second Yoga of Fulfillment workshop, Karen was vacationing with her family. Staying with friends, she happened upon an old issue of a magazine featuring an article about a town in the Midwest that was described as an ideal place to live and to raise a family. The article mentioned the excellence of its lower and middle school options. When Karen got home, she found the same magazine in her house; she had received it months earlier as part of a trial subscription offer. A few days later, a family member sent her a copy of the same article. "The universe was being very insistent," Karen told me.

Thus began Karen's odyssey, a sequence of events and "coincidences" that ultimately led to Karen fulfilling her goal.

In effect, one circumstance after another led to Karen and her family moving two thousand miles away to live in the town described in the magazine. Before doing so, they wound up selling their home, in a slow real estate market, for more than their asking price; in fact, it sold for the exact sum that Karen had decided would be the ideal amount to facilitate the move. (Hence her remark that the house has indeed "supported" them.) After selling that house, they purchased the home of their dreams—even though when they fell in love with it, it wasn't for sale. Last but not least, they enrolled their son in a school with the exact curriculum they had always wanted for him, but at a third of the price they would have had to pay had they remained in their old location.

Karen wanted to share her story with me in order to express her gratitude, and to affirm the value of the *Four Desires* process. Thanks to its methods and techniques, she had fulfilled her intentions not once but three different times: first with a successful renovation of her house and then with the sale of that house at a good price in a slow real estate market, thus enabling her to achieve her third goal, moving to a community that had all the characteristics she was longing for. In Karen's eyes, the steps of *The Four Desires* had not just helped her fulfill her desires, they had done so somewhat magically. "Both *sankalpas* I've drafted," she said, "have come true. Each time, it's been this effortless ride, a perfect series of events that one after another led to our dreams coming true."

Karen's portrayal of the effortlessness of fulfilling her intentions is not unfamiliar to me. I've heard it before. We all have. We've all read or heard about books, courses, and DVDs that promote the infinite power of intention, that say that if you focus on what you want and feel like you already have it, then all you have to do is step back and watch it manifest. Many of them portray a world in which there is no resistance to our achieving anything we want to achieve.

I had no problem accepting the idea that synchronicity played a part in Karen's fulfilling her desire. It usually does. However, having witnessed many people being successful with the same process and others being unsuccessful with it, I wasn't willing to attribute Karen's successes entirely to the phenomenon of synchronicity. So I probed a little deeper to get a clearer picture of exactly what role the *Four Desires* processes might have played. The more details I got, the less I was willing to credit the mysterious powers of intention and the more it confirmed my conviction that fulfilling our desires requires us to fully engage ourselves. Dreams do come true, but rarely without commitment and real effort.

> . . . .
> *If there is one thing that most often stands in the way of success, it's failing to make a thoughtful and continued effort to reach your "there."*
> . . . .

After Karen recounted all the events that had led her to "effortlessly" fulfill her desire, I asked for specifics about her commitment to the process. For example, how often did she work with her *sankalpa*? "All the time," she said matter-of-factly, and then, without pausing, she proceeded to tell me that she used to regularly eat bread or muffins several times a day. After discovering that she had an allergy to wheat products, she gave up the habit as her Departure Point. Giving up wheat provided her with many opportunities to work with Seed the Gap. "Oh, and I love Relax into Greatness. I do it every night along with my *sankalpa* when I go to sleep." She also mentioned the fact that although she did not meditate as much as she would have liked, she managed to do it for at least five minutes every morning before her children woke up. She also managed to do the Technique for Accessing Your *Dhi* (which I described in Chapter Seventeen) at least twice a week. Besides regularly practicing these steps, there was also the matter of her Dharma Code ("I receive Universal, loving guidance and channel it into the world with faith").

Karen had managed to formulate a Dharma Code that resonated deeply for her. Her commitment to it, even in the face of various challenges, was at the core of what led to her intention being fulfilled. By giving her a clear sense that she was being guided by a source of genuine wisdom, it gave her the confidence to navigate her way through selling their house for the price she wanted even when the experts, including her real estate agent, were pessimistic. More important, this confidence helped her find the courage to have an honest conversation with her mother about her desire to move, and it allowed her to discover that what her mother wanted most for Karen was not for her to remain geographically close but for her to stay emotionally close. Karen and her mother ended up feeling closer to each other than ever.

Karen's commitment to her Dharma Code was the real power that established her in a course of action that led to her family living a better life in their new community. Her openness to her inner guidance was responsible for many of the "coincidences" she'd mentioned. For example, when she went online to learn more about the town she'd read about, she found a link to a video of a couple in the town who had just gotten married, and for some reason she clicked on it and found herself watching the video. The ceremony touched her and left a strong impression. After surfing additional links, Karen's intuition told her to enter a raffle that was being held there. A few days later, a town resident named Paul called her about the raffle ticket she had bought. Although she hadn't won anything, she learned during the course of their conversation that Paul was the man whose wedding video she had watched a few days earlier. When she mentioned that she was considering moving there, Paul said that he and his wife would love to host Karen and her husband and show them around the town if they came to visit.

The joy Karen took in the process was also a significant part of her success. It was the grease that kept all the wheels turning. Put all the details of the picture together and it adds up to someone who played a very active role in the process rather than just deciding on an intention and waiting for the magic to unfold.

Karen's process, which culminated in her fulfilling her desires, began during the yoga courses, but it didn't end there. The workshops served as preparation for her continued commitment to the process, just as the work I've asked you to do throughout this book is your preparation. Before the end of every Yoga of Fulfillment workshop, I emphasize that, more often than not, the biggest difference between those who wind up having their dreams fulfilled and those who don't is what you do on a regular basis after the course is over.

It's not wrong to say that intention affects destiny. However, the point I've made throughout this book is that it *is* wrong to say that if you wish for things—even if you wish with great intensity—they will always materialize. The details of Karen's story demonstrate what I've observed generally to be the case: fulfilling your intention has less to do with the mysterious power of intention than with the wisdom contained in a well-known adage, "You reap what you sow." If there is one thing that most often stands in the way of success, it's failing to make a thoughtful and continued effort to reach your "there."

The Art of Practice

In the introduction, I wrote that to be successful with the *Four Desires* process it should be seen and approached as a practice. Now, as you near the end of learning about and working with the different steps of the process, it's useful to look more closely at what *practice* means.

In the *Yoga Sutras,* the Sanskrit term for practice is *abhyasa,* the literal meanings of which include "endeavor" or "repeat." However, practice, as the sage Patanjali makes clear, is not repetition for its own sake. He elaborates on what constitutes practice when he says that it is "the sustained effort to 'be there' or 'in that' (*tatra* in Sanskrit). Thus two key concepts define practice: "sustained effort" and "to 'be there.'" Sustained effort means that practice is necessarily done over time and consistently. This should not come as a great surprise. Whether you are trying to work your way into the Professional Golfers' Association, become a concert pianist, or master a particular yoga pose, you will need to work on the particular skill over and over again before you reach your "there."

In the context of the *Yoga Sutras,* Patanjali is using the term *there* to mean the goal of yoga: the stillness and mastery over one's mind that reveal the highest states of human experience. In the context of *The Four Desires,* your "there" is long-term happiness and prosperity. This includes fulfilling any one of your four desires that serves your long-term happiness. Thus, your practice entails being mindful of your goal while consistently endeavoring to reach it.

The *Yoga Sutras* tell us that for a practice to be effective, it must have three essential elements: it must be done for a long time, it must be done consistently, and it must be done with love or reverence. You don't have to look very hard to see that Karen's practice complied with Patanjali's guidelines for an effective practice. Being ever mindful of her goal and sustaining her effort over time, with consistency and with a love for the process, had everything to do with her achieving her goal.

Many people, despite being earnest and endeavoring to make a "sustained effort to be there," fail to do at least one necessary step in their practice. And they may not even realize it.

Teri's Story

My student Teri tried to change her circumstances for several years. She felt stuck, but it was not from a lack of motivation or effort. She had a *sankalpa,* which she repeated along with Relax into Greatness on a regular basis, and she meditated practically every day. Her *sankalpa* focused on writing a book for a major publisher. Although she was disciplined in her work, after two years of preparing various versions of a book proposal and trying to find a literary agent, the proposal had garnered little interest and no agent. She wasn't getting any closer to her "there."

At this point, Teri approached me for advice. After talking briefly, I had two words for her: Departure Point. The suggestion seemed to flip a switch. She immediately gave up her habit of endless news consumption (newspaper, television, Internet, blogs, you name it). Results came quickly.

Two months later, Teri had a new proposal and an agent. She attributed the dra-

> . . . .
> *Whoever said "Practice makes perfect" was half right; practice does make perfect—if you are doing the right practice.*
> . . . .

matic turn of events to using her news media fast to effectively seed the gap with her resolution. This practice, she said, infused her with a powerful wave of optimism and catalyzed ideas. The right practice made all the difference, transforming her outlook and allowing her to be in the right place at the right time to attract the right agent.

Teri had taken a gigantic leap toward her intention by implementing the practical step of finding the one element of the *Four Desires* process that she had previously neglected and then incorporating it into her practice. By putting my advice into action, Teri wrote differently, felt differently about her writing and herself, and presented herself and her book differently to the agents she met.

Whoever said "Practice makes perfect" was half right; practice does make perfect—if you are doing the right practice. If you are doing the wrong one or you are doing a practice that is incomplete, the amount of effort you are applying to it may not matter. As we've seen, "sustained effort" (Patanjali's term) is crucial to increasing the likelihood of achieving your dreams, but sustained effort has to be applied correctly.

It would be convenient if there were a single fix for everyone who has run aground before fulfilling his or her desire. Unfortunately, there are many answers. We are all different and want different things. We all want what we want with different levels of intensity. We all have different levels and kinds of internal and external resistance, and we all have different ways of responding to the resistance we face.

It may be that the foundation for your practice needs to be stronger—which would mean refining your Dharma Code. It may be that practicing Relax into Greatness more regularly could make a significant difference or that committing to seeing things from your Miracle Angle could be the key. The most common reason for not fulfilling a goal is probably a lack of sustained effort: many people just give up too soon. If you find yourself struggling, how do you figure out which step you need to focus on, which part of the process you need to improve upon or engage in more frequently to fulfill your desire? The coming chapters are dedicated to helping you answer this vital question.

CHAPTER 25

. . . .

NO ADJUSTMENT,
NO FULFILLMENT

Two underlying principles have been the basis for every step in this book. In this chapter, we will explore these principles and see how they are woven throughout the process of *The Four Desires*. In fact, these two principles help illuminate the ideal approach to living. You might say that they are the keys to solving any and all of life's challenges.

Swami Rama often talked about these two principles, which he called *adjustment* and *contentment,* as the "secret to living in the external world." Together, they are the "how" for endeavoring to reach your "there."

Contentment is peace. It is the result of abiding in the truth of who you are. It is the gift that unfolds as you glimpse that part of you that is free from suffering and disease at every level, the part of you that is limitless. The texts and teachers from all religious and spiritual traditions remind us

> . . . .
>
> *To the degree that we master contentment, it is possible to find at least some measure of peace and acceptance in the midst of even the most intense hardships.*
>
> . . . .

time and time again that not only does such a part of you exist, but that lasting happiness depends on your finding it.

According to the yoga tradition, you access contentment through meditation (or through whatever process enables your mind to settle into an experience of timelessness). The experience of contentment gradually leads you to know that beyond your experiences and responses in the transitory world there is a part of you that is always at ease. In Spirit's abode, you have nothing to gain; you cannot be improved upon. You are what the Vedas describe as *tat tvam asi,* one with the Source—God, Essence—whole and complete just as you are.

Contentment affords you life's only real and lasting comfort. Resting in it, even in small measure, teaches you that while asserting yourself in the world is necessary for material pleasure and success, you are never really completely *of* the world. To the degree that we master contentment, it is possible to find at least some measure of peace and acceptance in the midst of even the most intense hardships. This means that solace, inspiration, and the taste of fulfillment are always accessible.

Developing contentment is the primary intention behind all the meditations found in this book. It is an integral part of what allowed you, through the Bliss Meditation, to uncover your *sankalpa* and to access your *dhi.* Relax into Greatness is another door to contentment, allowing you to bask in the feeling of having already achieved your *sankalpa,* and in so doing, imbuing your unconscious with a sense of direction to help you achieve it. Contentment is also vital to the most pivotal step of the process, *vairagya.* Accessing contentment through meditation allows you to apply non-attachment to any situation more easily. Throughout the course of your life, the more you access contentment, the more likely it is that you'll rise to the higher stages of non-attachment and acceptance.

There will be times, however, when sitting quietly and delighting in the treasures of the Infinite will not lead you toward either lasting or short-term happiness. At such times, you have to refine your relationships (to yourself, to others, or to things in your life) if you are to continue to respond to Spirit's grand scheme or *dharma.* In other words, at such times adjustment is required.

The well-being of every organism is directly related to its capacity to adjust. For example, stress is a call to adjust your attitude about what is causing the stress, your actions, or both. In this sense, stress can actually be helpful, since it is a call to adjust in order to improve. Illness can also be a call for adjustment. Hypertension, for example, which is called "the silent killer," kills approximately forty thousand Americans every year, but most of these deaths would be preventable if those who had the disease would adjust their diets and their exercise regimes. Adjustment, however, does more than just ensure your survival; it is the basis of thriving.

Adjustment can be internal, external, or both. Internal adjustment relates to changing your attitudes, expectations, beliefs, judgments, or attachments. External adjustment consists of creating real or material changes in the way you act or in your circumstances. This means your habits, including how you spend your time and your money, how you treat other people, and how you treat yourself. Adjustment could involve spending less time on things that are unimportant and becoming more attentive to the things that matter. It could mean taking a walk after dinner or meditating on a regular basis; it could entail changing the foods that you eat, how often you work out, how many hours per day you work, how organized you are, even how you prepare for bed.

Adjustment might result in your becoming more productive, understanding, effective, peaceful, alert, prosperous, kind, generous, thoughtful, disciplined, and active; becoming healthier; or developing one of countless other qualities that support your growth and development.

Adjustment is the basis of Departure Point, the deliberate action of giving up a habit and seeding the gap with your intention. Adjustment enables you to adjust the level of intensity of your desire and act on the power to do what you know. Adjustment is also the basis for releasing your Grievance Angle, finding your Miracle Angle, and then taking appropriate action based on it.

> . . . .
> *Adjustment, however, does more than just ensure your survival; it is the basis of thriving.*
> . . . .

The key, of course, is not just to *think* about adjustment but to *do* it. You can contemplate doing the exercises in this book, joining a health club, stopping smoking, or going to couples counseling, but as we've seen, until you actually set into motion one of the actions that would make your life better, you should not expect much improvement.

This is why I say "No adjustment, no fulfillment."

Claudia's Story

Claudia had studied yoga with me over the years and had friends who had taken the Yoga of Fulfillment workshop and briefed her on it, but she'd never taken the course herself. When she discovered I would be traveling to the city where she lived, she e-mailed my office to ask if I'd meet with her to talk about her struggles to achieve her goal. When we sat down to talk, I learned that her knowledge of the process was far from complete. She thought *The Four Desires* consisted of just finding a *sankalpa* and practicing Relax into Greatness, both of which she had been doing for over a year. "A lot of amazing things happened the first month or so that I was doing them," she told me, "but then nothing really came of it." She wanted me to tell her why.

Claudia was a special-needs teacher at a prestigious private school on the west coast. She was adored by the children she worked with and respected by their parents. However, Claudia was frustrated with her job. Repeated policy changes at the school were making it increasingly difficult for her to continue to use the methods and approaches that she and the parents of the children with whom she worked knew to have the most positive impact on her students. Over the years, Claudia's frustration had grown, and she decided she wanted to start her own school and name it the Children's Center for Creative Development. Her *sankalpa* was: "The Children's Center for Creative Development is thriving and supporting the community it was built to serve."

Within just a few weeks of working with this *sankalpa* and practicing Relax into Greatness, some parents approached Claudia—with no solicitation on her part—to tell her that if she was interested in opening and supervising a school for children with special needs, they were prepared to back her financially. Claudia was elated. Everything seemed to be working wonderfully; her *sankalpa* had created an opportunity that seemed as if it would soon help manifest her dream. But now, twelve months later, the Children's Center for Creative Development had not materialized.

I asked Claudia if she knew why nothing had come from that initial wave of enthusiasm and support. Her immediate response was, "Confidence." The parents had pulled back, she reasoned, because she didn't exude enough of it; because of her lack of confidence, they had lost confidence in her. "Yup, it's basically a lack of confidence. You got anything for that?" she quipped.

Before I could answer her, Claudia quickly and flippantly began to explain why the parents' lack of confidence was justified. Speaking quickly, she reeled off a list of all the things she would have been incapable of: fund-raising, creating a start-up budget, commissioning design plans, acquiring permits, writing contracts for administrators and teachers . . .

As she spoke, I found myself paying less attention to what she was saying and more and more to the manner in which she said it. Claudia had a way of constantly dismissing both herself and the things she cared about most. The more she cared about something, the less important she made it sound. Along the way she used humor to undercut herself even more, to the point that it was tempting not to take seriously anything she said. But I sensed that beneath the veneer of flippancy, she cared deeply about her vocation, even if she was conflicted about it and even less clear about how to move forward in her life. I decided I needed to be direct with her.

"Claudia," I said, "how easy is it for you to admit what you want?" Her blank stare told me she hadn't expected the question. I followed it with two others: "I have to ask, do you value what you do? And if so, how much?"

"Kind of . . . barely. I don't know. Why?"

"Because when you spoke about running the center, you didn't sound insecure, you sounded detached, as though if it didn't happen it wouldn't make much difference to you. Would it?"

"Yes . . . no. What should I say? What's the right answer?"

"You tell me, Claudia. But if that's how you responded to the parents who were prepared to back you and who looked to you to lead the project, I'm not surprised they eventually lost interest."

"Okay," she said warily.

"You came to me because you said you wanted help manifesting this school. Do you?"

She nodded.

"Then why is it so hard for you to be excited about it?"

She shrugged. "Don't know."

"In the same breath you say you'd love to do it and that it's your dream, then you practically dismiss its value altogether. Like you could take or leave the whole thing."

"You're right," she said, her demeanor suddenly changing. "It's just that it's hard for me to admit how much I want it, for fear that if I don't get it I'll feel like even more of a failure."

Now we were getting somewhere. "Do you want to see the center happen?"

"Yeah, sure I do. I think so . . . I'm sorry. Yes, I do. Definitely."

"Then why are you so focused on the possibility of failure instead of success?"

"Owning my worth and embracing the things I really want, it's . . . it's always been a struggle. It's one of my biggest challenges. It's why I don't charge enough for what I do. In my marriage, in everything, it's always been practically impossible for me to admit—to myself and others—what I really want or that I deserve it."

"Claudia, a lot of what we're really talking about is related to self-worth. It's important that you take a look at whether or not you believe you're worthy of having what you want. If you believe you are, then stop apologizing for your desires and for what matters most to you. What you want could be of extraordinary value. You have value, inherently, and as a teacher, you're valuable too. If this school happened, it would be of great value to the kids you teach and to their parents. Everyone seems to be able to admit that except you."

"That makes sense," she acknowledged.

"So, one more time, do you want the center to happen?"

"Yes."

"Then you need to put your fears aside and act like it. If self-worth has been a challenge for you, then you need a Dharma Code to address it. If the school is going to happen, it's essential that you embrace your own value as well as the center's."

She let out a big sigh. "Yup."

"Claudia, your missing key is adjustment. You have to change. Before things can change, *you* have to. It's up to you. If you powerfully believe in the value of what you offer the world, your love and passion for it will become an unstoppable force. Then you will attract things commensurate to that force. People and opportunities will come forward that will support your conviction and make it more likely that your desire will come to fruition."

Claudia agreed. We then talked about how she could build her self-worth. I gave her some specific techniques that I thought would help. I asked her to start a daily meditation practice again, specifically the practice I shared in Chapter Twelve (Meditation to Increase *Shakti*), at the end of which she was to rest in deep feelings of self-worth, a state easily accessed with a still mind. I also asked her to identify her *vikalpa*—the contrary desire that had been acting against her stated desire. I gave her the *vikalpa* exercise in Chapter Thirteen to help her see both the internal and external resistances that stood in her way. I asked her to do Relax into Greatness to help her develop more capacity to let go and to build her dispassion. I emphatically reminded her that nothing was more vital than for her to uncover her Dharma Code. I wanted to help Claudia get past her doubts and insecurities and become committed to a Dharma Code that would help her to become a force of Nature. She needed to identify her purpose, her life lesson—what she was meant to live for in a larger sense, even beyond the center.

By the end of the conversation, Claudia was inspired and confident. We both felt her enthusiasm about the work I'd asked her to do. She seemed ready and willing to create a new path for herself. We agreed that in a month or two she would e-mail me to let me know how things were going. She assured me she would soon have the center back on track.

For the next year, Claudia didn't contact me. Not until I ran into her did I learn that the center was exactly where it had been when we had last spoken. Not surprisingly, Claudia was too. "Personal things came up that needed my attention and I kind of lost interest in the whole thing," she said. I asked if she had done her homework. Instead of answering directly, she told me how full her teaching schedule was. I didn't press any further. I would have offered her some advice, but she hadn't asked for any, and she seemed embarrassed, eager for our conversation to be over. And before I could think of anything else to say, she was saying goodbye. As she turned to leave, she added, "There's always next lifetime, right?"

It would be easy to underestimate the magnitude of the work I had asked Claudia to do and to leap to a negative judgment of her. I didn't see it that way. I understood that for her to achieve her dreams meant that she would have had to confront—and make the commitment to disengage from—deep, long-standing patterns. It was no surprise that she had resistance; unfortunately, her resistance had won.

Claudia's story is particularly relevant as a contrast with Karen's. I knew, and had told Claudia so a year earlier, that unless she herself changed, the chances of her fulfilling her dream were practically nil. No adjustment, no fulfillment. Karen, unlike Claudia, did adjust. To fulfill her desire to live in the right community for her family, Karen worked to uncover her *vikalpa,* her own inner conflict, and once she recognized it she moved to resolve it by having a conversation with her mother. When they sat down to talk, she came to the realization that in following her long-standing habit of trying to please her mother, she had been assuming—wrongly—that she knew what her mother wanted. This was very freeing. Karen also gathered her resources, and when the time was right to make the move to another state that was the key to fulfilling her desire, she sold her home and moved there. I'd like to be able to say that when given a clear choice to go the way of Karen and choose adjustment, most people make that choice, but the truth is that more often than not, they don't. Claudia is only one of hundreds if not thousands of people I've watched who, for any number of reasons, failed to adjust.

Steven's Story

When I first met Steven, he was in his early sixties, and despite exercising regularly, he had a long list of ailments that he hoped yoga could alleviate: chronic insomnia, headaches, lower back problems, shortness of breath, and almost constant pain from muscular tension in his neck and shoulders.

The first time I taught him I led him through a yoga practice specifically tailored to treat his symptoms. Afterward, he felt markedly better. I told him I believed that if he regularly practiced yoga, proper breathing techniques, relaxation, and meditation, it was likely that he would greatly improve his health. I left our session with both of us believing that if he applied himself, he'd fulfill his wish.

Steven asked me to design a practice for him. He hired me to lead him through it at least once a week to make sure he was doing it correctly and to modify the program as I saw fit. The other six days he practiced it on his own. A month later, he'd made significant progress. But soon afterward, I observed an alarming pattern, one that made it all but impossible for Steven to fulfill his desire for better health.

At least once a month, Steven would go out of town for a few days, during which he didn't practice at all. These few days away from home would debilitate him. Not only did the worst of his symptoms return, but when he came back I would have to walk him through the most basic elements of his practice as if he had never done it before. I'd never seen anything quite like it. How could just a few days of not practicing have such a negative effect? Eventually I learned what was causing the problem.

During his trips out of town, Steven would use drugs (marijuana, cocaine, and I'm not sure what else). The effects of these binge weekends were devastating on his aging body. Time and again, whatever progress his yoga practice provided was nullified by his drug-binge lifestyle.

In the early days, I hoped that our work together could make enough of a difference that he would no longer want to do the things that were having such a detrimental effect on him. Unfortunately, this never happened. Months passed, then years. Nothing changed.

Steven's desire to be healthier was attainable, but it could never happen without his making real changes. In my eyes, Steven, who in material terms was a powerful and successful man, came to represent a cautionary tale about the pivotal role that adjustment plays in determining just how much we will thrive in our lifetime. Steven showed me that no matter how capable we are, no matter how much we've achieved, how accomplished we become at yoga postures, how slow and smooth our breath might be, or how much contentment we access through meditation and relaxation, without the right adjustment it may all be worthless. When it comes to fulfilling our intention, adjustment can make or break our chances of having what we really want.

Denise's Story

Denise wanted to be married. More than anything, she longed for a husband with whom she could raise a family. She had a successful career, which she enjoyed, but no amount of career advancement ever truly fulfilled her, because what she really wanted kept eluding her.

Attractive, healthy, and bright, Denise traveled the world. She was stylish and had a good sense of humor. Men were attracted to her and she had relationships. Yet although she attracted men interested in long-term relationships, her relationships with them never seemed to last.

At one point she confided to me that with the failure of each relationship, her anger and frustration about men (and life in general) grew. Over the years it was hard not to notice her becoming increasingly bitter. On the surface, she was full of exuberance, busy with life and work. As she approached her late thirties, Denise's outward appearance of joyfulness had become as much a coping mechanism as a way of exhibiting to the world what she would like to feel. If you didn't know her well and didn't look too closely, she might have seemed like an incredibly fun person to be around, but once you got close, you saw that despite her carefree personality, she was anything but. I suspect that sooner or later Denise projected her unresolved resentments onto the men she was dating, and they ended up breaking it off with her because they could sense that anger.

In the almost ten years I taught her, Denise never made an adjustment. I watched this take its toll on her and on the likelihood of her having a long-term relationship. What was once a small irritation with men grew to the point where a part of her now seemed to barely tolerate them. It made little difference if they were male supervisors at work, past lovers, her two brothers (each of whom was married with kids), or a new man who became interested in her. Denise had settled into a difficult predicament: the very thing she hoped to attract was the focus of a lot of anger and frustration.

My last opportunity to help her adjust was at a Yoga of Fulfillment workshop I taught five years ago. Denise had framed her *sankalpa* around her desire for a lasting relationship: "I'm married to the man of my dreams and we're expecting our first child." At one point during the workshop, I asked if I could see her *vikalpa* exercise. I was surprised to see that there was not a single mention of her conflicted feelings about relationships, so I asked her directly whether she might have any residual feelings of negativity toward men in general or any one man in particular. I asked her as discreetly as possible, aware that I was a man who was asking her to examine her difficulties in dealing with one of my own kind.

Denise responded calmly, saying, "No, but I'll think about it." She was cordial, but I knew I had hit a nerve. During the rest of the course she was disengaged, barely willing to do the remaining exercises. The truth is she chose to stop being my student at that moment and has never studied with me again.

It's not important whether or not Denise remained my student. No teacher can be a good match for every student, and that's often neither the teacher's fault nor the student's. If her next teacher had managed to help her get closer to having what she wanted, I would be only too pleased. But it's now been more than five years, and through mutual friends I know that Denise is still searching for a man, still wanting a long-term relationship.

Initially, at least, it wasn't hard to inspire Claudia, Steven, or Denise. Yet none of them did what needed to be done to get closer to fulfilling their desires. Nothing was more fundamental in preventing them from getting what they wanted than *not* doing the work of adjustment.

CHAPTER 26

THE PAIN OF NOT CHANGING

Over the years, I've lectured to tens of thousands of people on the subject of improving the quality of their lives. An essential element of doing so is spending at least some time each day in solitude and learning to clear and quiet the mind. I speak from my experience as a teacher, someone who has seen the countless ways that stress negatively impacts people's lives. I also speak from my experience as a father of four children, a husband, and a business owner. I have felt, as well as seen in others, the powerful and profound difference that even a little time for solitude and a clear and quiet mind can make in your life.

After I describe the physiological, emotional, mental, and of course spiritual benefits of taking even just a few minutes a day to do a meditation or relaxation practice, I notice that most people seem inspired to do it, but I've also observed that only a small percentage ever act on the inspiration. Why? The simple answer is pain. It's all about pain.

More than three decades ago, I was just beginning to try to establish a regular meditation practice. Almost instantly, meditation helped me feel and think noticeably better. I still recall how much those first days of practicing stirred in me a sense of limitless possibility and of what life might be like if I practiced meditation consistently. Not long after I began to experience its benefits, I also discovered that there were times I would resist doing it. Curious about how to convert my enthusiasm for it into a regular practice and overcome my resistance, I approached my teacher.

"Remember what it feels like when you don't do it," he suggested. Sensing my confusion, he asked, "What does it feel like when you miss a day?"

"Not good," I said. "I feel less clear, less inspired, less confident, less comfortable."

"Put that at the forefront of your mind," he told me. "The more you remain clear about the pain of not doing it, the less likely you are to miss a day of practice."

As odd as it sounded to me at the time, I soon realized he was right, and that the reason this insight is so accurate has to do with the psychology of initiating a new behavior.

Clinical research has shown that in the early stages of trying to form a new behavior or habit, the benefits the new habit will afford us, no matter how powerful they are, are often outweighed by the desire to avoid the pain of change. This is the approach/avoidance conundrum. Claudia, for example, wanted to approach opening her special-needs school, but part of her also wanted to avoid having to adjust and confront her problems with self-worth in order to see that dream fulfilled. In short, the pull or attraction of her desire to be the founder of a new school was less powerful than her desire to avoid the feelings and issues that she found painful.

Claudia's conflict, her vacillation between approach and avoidance, is not unusual. Research has shown that most of the time "the tendency to avoid is stronger than the tendency to approach." In other words, often we behave in ways that are counterproductive in order to avoid the effort—the immediate pain—involved in change, even though in doing so we are aware that we are causing ourselves long-term pain. An addict, for example, despite inflicting no small measure of suffering on himself, won't stop using drugs or alcohol as long as it seems harder to stop than to continue. That's why so many addicts are finally able to stop only when they hit their "bottom"—when at last it is clear to them that the pain of continuing is greater than the pain of stopping.

In a sense, we all run the risk of being addicted to the feelings, beliefs, and behaviors we have grown used to. As long as you identify change as being more painful than not changing, the odds are that you won't. For example, if you want to lose weight but you haven't shifted your perception enough to realize that changing your diet and increasing the amount you exercise is less painful than continuing to be overweight, it is unlikely that you will really commit to losing weight. That's why some people finally lose weight only when a doctor tells them that they are in imminent danger of developing diabetes, or having a stroke, or suffering a heart attack if they don't.

However, psychologists report that if, as time goes on, you experience enough of the benefits of the new behavior that you've been struggling to commit to, the balance tips in favor of that behavior. In other words, once a habit has been established and you've started to reap its rewards, pleasure replaces pain as your main motivating factor.

Unfortunately, doing something new, even something that you want to do and that you know will be good for you, may not feel good right away. Psychological studies show that the power of pleasure usually manifests relatively late in the process of trying to form a new behavior. It is worth noting, however, that instilling new and positive associations into the unconscious, through the regular practice of Relax into Greatness in combination with *sankalpa,* can help speed up this transition and make it easier to establish new patterns of behavior.

In my case, Mani's advice came at just the right time, when the pleasure of meditating was already strong enough to enable me to shift my motivation from avoiding pain (the pain of making a change) to finding pleasure. After several weeks of reaping the benefits and pleasures of meditation, I quickly learned that not meditating was more unpleasant than the effort required to put aside the time for it, and I stopped resisting altogether. At this point, nearly three decades later, I relish the time I spend in meditation. With little or no effort, I do it every day. My longing for the positive feelings meditation provides is all the motivation I need to keep doing it.

That said, it does take a while to get to the point where pleasure becomes your dominant motivation. Humankind has long understood that the threat of pain is a more immediately effective stimulus for creating a desired behavior. For example, when you are caught driving over the speed limit, you get a ticket and a fine; you do not get a thank-you note and a bouquet of flowers each time you *don't* speed.

The same reasoning pervades most spiritual traditions. It's no accident that many religious and even spiritual traditions spell out the repercussions of not heeding the teachings: suffering, damnation, hell, the final judgment, purgatory, and the like. These dire warnings are usually contrasted with the promise of *nirvana,* salvation, heaven, enlightenment, God's good graces, liberation, and bliss if one does follow the teachings. Unfortunately, while we are somewhat motivated by the promise of the benefits we stand to reap, the threat of fire and brimstone is usually more effective at getting us to change.

Stop for a moment and consider the implications. Throughout *The Four Desires,* I've asked you to do certain exercises and practices to help you improve the quality of your life. Did you do all of them? Did you do some of them? Did you do any of them? How completely have you embraced adjustment? How much are you going to adjust after you've finished reading this book?

Which is greater, the pain of not having what you want or the pain of making the changes necessary to getting it? How can you tell which is greater?

One way of telling which pain is greater to you at this moment is to survey the symptoms. If you haven't completed all of the exercises I've asked you to do, if you've backpedaled on your commitments (including your commitment to take care of yourself) or resumed the habit that you pledged to stop as your Departure Point, if you haven't responded to your inner wisdom (or not even sought it for guidance), if you haven't started or maintained a regular meditation or relaxation process even though a part of you longs for it, it is a sign that you associate more pain with changing than you do with not fulfilling your intention.

Know the Consequences

Each time I lead a seminar on the principles of *The Four Desires,* I ask the participants to do one final exercise in which they will write about the cost of not applying what they have learned. This is my last opportunity to instill a sense of the critical role their own commitment and effort will play in influencing their success or failure in attaining their goals. It's important that I acknowledge, and that they leave the course expecting, that sooner or later they will encounter resistance. Before they start this last exercise, I paint as clear a picture of the stakes as I can, giving them a general sense of the price of their not adjusting and, therefore, not attaining the lasting happiness their souls seek.

What I tell them is this: "Tomorrow the course will be over and you'll be headed home. At some time in the future, some of you will have achieved your desires. Some of you will not. The biggest factor in determining which of the two it will be is *you*—or, more specifically, the actions you do or do not take. It's important that you are clear about what will motivate you to act one way or the other. What will inspire you enough to change and to do what is necessary to achieve or to become what you want? The answer may surprise you. In most cases it's not the power of your dream. Rather, it's the pain of coming face-to-face with not achieving your goal, of realizing how easy it is to let the opportunity for doing so slip through your fingers.

> . . . .
>
> *Don't postpone your happiness. The best time to take stock of your life is long before some tragedy touches you to confirm that life doesn't last forever.*
>
> . . . .

" 'There are two pains in life: the pain of discipline and the pain of regret. We each choose which of the two we will suffer.' " This is an anonymous quote commonly invoked by coaches in the sports world. The problem is that in life you are not always paying attention to the scoreboard, and even if you are, there's a good chance you are not watching the clock.

Once in a while, however, you do look at the clock. You stare at it in disbelief, amazed at how much time has passed while you were not paying attention. It is now gone forever. One day it will run out completely. Think of the last time you attended a funeral. Did it remind you of just how fragile and temporary life is? You probably left the service telling yourself that you will now start living with a sense of the urgency of time. You committed yourself then and there, because some part of you knew that if you did anything less, you would be squandering the gift of life with which you have been blessed.

The best way to ensure that you live fully is to be aware that you are not going to live forever. There are many causes of pain in life, but keep this in mind: the pain of not doing, not honoring your soul's call, may well exceed all others. Dying without having lived the fullest life possible is the worst pain.

The point is, don't postpone your happiness. The best time to take stock of your life is long before some tragedy touches you to confirm that life doesn't last forever.

It may be uncomfortable to hear that the difference between having what you desire and not having it depends on whether or not you allow yourself to fully acknowledge the pain of not changing, but that does not change the fact that it invariably does.

The question you need to ask yourself is, how bad does it have to feel before you are motivated to act differently and effect real change in your life? You can decide today that the price of not changing is too high, and that you refuse to stay just as you are. It's up to you.

This is the terrain not just of the following exercise, but of your life. Now it is time for you to turn your attention to the consequences of not following through and doing what you need to do to achieve your goals.

EXERCISE: KNOW THE CONSEQUENCES

To the extent that a part of you wants to avoid what happened to Claudia, Steven, and Denise, then it's vital for you to do this exercise.

You'll need a pen or pencil and two sheets of paper.

Take ten minutes to write about the consequences, including the emotional, financial, physical, and spiritual pain, of your desire not being fulfilled. Your assignment is to identify the cost of not following through, of not taking the actions that would move you toward achieving the life you want. Write about the specific impact on you and on your life if you do not make the necessary changes, or if you fail to apply or continue applying any of the specific steps in *The Four Desires*. What are the ways you will suffer?

The point of the exercise is to make the consequences of not having what you want palpable enough that you will be motivated to make the necessary adjustment. Spelling out the consequences in writing will support your decision that this time will be different from all the other times when you wanted to take control of your life but stopped short of doing it.

Now that you've done this exercise, you possess an essential motivational tool to empower you to commit to your endeavor indefinitely. It's crucial to point out, however, that just because you've identified the consequences of not following through doesn't necessarily mean that they will remain foremost in your mind when resistance comes up. When you recognize the symptoms of resistance, you may have to deliberately recall what you wrote about the consequences of giving in to it. It will be up to you to decide if and when you need to remind yourself of these consequences. On the other hand, if you find yourself implementing change despite possible resistance, it is a sure sign that you are aware of the cost of not fulfilling your desires—and that, unlike Claudia, you are not operating on the expectation that there will be a "next lifetime" in which to achieve them.

The need to adjust, and all that it entails, is never done. Life is constantly changing, and so must we. However, having made the case for "no adjustment, no fulfillment," I think it is important to again acknowledge that there will be times where no amount of action or adjustment—no matter how right—will resolve all our challenges and fulfill all our needs. Try as we might, our efforts at deliberate change will not always provide us with the happiness that we are seeking. For that reason there is contentment. Let's turn our attention to it.

. . . .

CHAPTER 27

CONTENTMENT CHANGES
EVERYTHING

By most measures, Deborah had it all: three healthy, beautiful children, a loving and faithful husband whose income supported them and provided the family with a lovely home and an abundant life. They were able to take family vacations twice a year, and Deborah could afford to update her wardrobe on a regular basis. They had all the latest appliances, nice cars—basically, whatever they wanted. Deborah had the luxury of being free to do whatever she chose to do with her time. She was a dedicated mother, blessed with a magnetic, vibrant personality. She was beloved and treasured by her close friends.

Yet as ideal as her life may have appeared on the outside, inside Deborah felt uneasy. She lived with persistent frustration and no clear sense of how to resolve it. Despite being able to afford to satisfy most of her material wants, she lived with a nagging sense of disappointment—"if only life were different." If only her husband had more time for her or her kids listened more, or just maybe if she could go back to the life she had before kids and a husband, the nagging sense of dissatisfaction would be lifted.

Deborah never considered this last one as a real option, but she often fantasized about the many things that might solve her predicament. She also tried different things in the hope of finding her solution: shopping, massage, therapy, dieting, yoga, photography classes, greater involvement in her kids' school. She turned to several self-help books. She searched out everything she could think of, save the one that would wind up making the difference—contentment.

Deborah had known about meditation for years. The last minute or two of the yoga classes she attended usually ended with it, but because it was her least favorite part of class, she never thought of devoting time to it outside class. However, one day, while trying to sit still during meditation at the end of class, she felt something new, a kind of wholeness that she had never experienced before. She had an epiphany. She approached her teacher, a student of mine, and asked for some guidance to practice meditation at home. Suzanne recommended that she meditate on her breath and gave her simple directions for practicing it. She emphasized that Deborah should do the practice consistently for forty days, irrespective of the results. "Even if you only do it for five minutes, do it every day," Suzanne told her.

The first day at home, Deborah did her best to sit still and simply follow her breath. It sounded so ridiculously simple: "Follow your breath." But it wasn't as simple as it sounded. "Why should something that is so simple be so hard?" She was intrigued. She decided that she was up for the challenge and that there would be something to gain from learning to get her mind to be more still.

The first month, Deborah managed to meditate five or six days a week, on average for nearly twenty minutes each time. It took a while, but as time went on she experienced that her body and mind were fighting it less and less. At some point she actually began to enjoy the process and looked forward to doing it.

Deborah had decided not to tell anyone that she was going to start practicing meditation; she didn't want others' expectations of her to influence her. Yet within a couple of weeks of starting her practice, she heard from several friends that she seemed different, more at ease. Her husband mentioned that there was something lighter and more playful about her. None of these comments surprised her; Deborah hadn't felt so inspired for as long as she could remember.

Weeks followed during which her time in meditation seemed to fly by. But then, just when she was feeling that she had overcome the hard part, she hit a period where meditating seemed harder than ever. For the next month or two, her practice would vary from being effortless and calm to being very uncomfortable. It took some additional support and guidance from Suzanne for Deborah to meet the challenges of sitting through her restlessness and resistance and to continue practicing. But she did.

Then one day she had a powerful, life-changing insight. The mood of dissatisfaction that had long been part of her life, she realized, was not so much a part of *her* as it was something that, at some level, she was choosing to hold on to. Her chronic dissatisfaction was suddenly no more real to her than a dream, one that she had been dreaming for far too long. Suddenly she felt herself "wake up," completely unidentified with the old dream.

A few months after she began meditating, the feelings that had plagued Deborah for years had lifted almost entirely. The result was that her expectations of her life and family changed. The aimlessness that used to define her had become a thing of the past. She now sought friends and activities that seemed essential to her, and she spent less time on things that were unimportant to her. She began taking better care of herself, exercising regularly, and spending more time with the friends she really respected, and she also returned to photography, a long-lost love. To her surprise, taking time out of her busy life to meditate was helping her find more time and better ways to enjoy it. She was doing more of what mattered most to her, but accomplishing more was not the *source* of her happiness; it was the *result* of it. Deborah's newfound joy had nothing to do with achievement. Her life had changed thanks to her experiencing a greater measure of contentment.

> . . . .
> *You cannot think your way to an authentic version of contentment.*
> . . . .

It's not very difficult to find a temporary solution to the things that trouble you. From virtual shopping malls to the latest gossip magazines, you have countless diversions at your disposal. Any of them can gratify your fleeting wants, but none of them will ever fulfill your needs, the deeper longings that your soul is prompting you to fulfill. At the root of those longings is your soul's fourth desire, *moksha,* the desire for freedom or liberation. Contentment is the only thing that can provide it.

By starting and maintaining a regular meditation practice, Deborah found that she did not need to change her outer circumstances to experience fulfillment; the change she needed to make was internal. She needed to experience the contentment that was always there within her, available to her if only she could connect to it. But in order to experience contentment, she did need to make one external adjustment: she needed to consistently set aside the time to meditate.

Deborah's former malaise was a symptom, an indication of her need for the elixir of contentment, something her exciting, busy, and materially abundant life was unable to provide. Deborah is a case in point that to the degree that we lack contentment, even a life teeming with worldly riches and gratifications can be insufficiently fulfilling or meaningful. Precisely because she had become ensnared in her world of change, Deborah fell prey to a mild kind of helplessness. Meditation trained her to steady her mind enough to see the Source of life in all its glory and to recognize that the inner joy, the joy she had been searching for, is always present. Through meditation, Deborah learned to create the conditions necessary to experience it.

"This self is neither far or near; it is not inaccessible nor is it in distant places: it is what in oneself appears to be the experience of bliss, and is therefore realized in oneself." I cited this quote from the *Yoga Vasistha* earlier. It portrays Deborah's transformation perfectly. She searched far and wide, but all along she was actually seeking what only a vision of her self could provide. Nothing else would satisfy her need and resolve her discomfort. Only through the discipline of meditation could this have happened. Unfortunately, modern technology cannot provide any shortcuts to learning to still your mind.

Meditation, self-reflection, and contemplation are the methods prescribed by the ancient traditions to access contentment. Before it can be experienced, a seeker must first loosen his or her attachment to finite perception; thus identification with time, body, job, gender, and responsibilities as well as disappointment, jealousy, frustration, and the like must give way so that you can return to contentment. This letting go must be repeated each time before you can taste the sweetness of silence or reach the blissful realms of self-awareness beyond good and bad and the limits of mind.

I want to stress that contentment cannot be forced. It is not an attitude; it is not something you can convince yourself to feel. You cannot think your way to an authentic version of contentment, and it is not healthy or helpful to pretend that you are content when you are not. Yes, part of you is always free, joyous, and unconditionally at peace, but if this is just an idea to you, your only choice is to do the practices that will actually anchor you in the feelings and awareness found in contentment.

The Process of Contentment

Forcing yourself to act content when you are not genuinely so leads to all sorts of difficulty, conflict, and turmoil. Remember, contentment is a process, not a pill that can be ingested to produce instantaneous results. Even the best techniques and practices done correctly do not necessarily provide you instantly with the feelings for which you may be searching. In your first meditations, peace may be elusive. You may not experience contentment right away, or if you do experience it while in the practice, it may take a while—sometimes a long while—to pervade your life. This is especially true if you've waited a long time to start your practice. Remember, an effective practice is defined by repetition.

Throughout this book, in nearly every chapter, I've provided you with various methods for accessing contentment, any one of which would be ideal for you to work with. Do the one that attracts you. It should be the one that you enjoy most or the one that seems to best address your needs or aspirations. Once you've selected a practice, do it consistently for an extended period of time, and do it with respect and love. Trust that your practice will eventually bear the fruits of contentment, non-attachment, and freedom. Although the most profound results will probably take a while to develop, doing the right practice even a few times should provide you with some benefits sooner rather than later.

As Deborah's story makes clear, a life without contentment, without some measure of *moksha,* renders you blind to life's real treasures and the source of your suffering. Shelly's story is a powerful follow-up to Deborah's. It is a story about contentment, and about the power of the Healing the Heart Meditation that I walked you through earlier.

It had been a demanding week. I'd just finished teaching a seminar and said my goodbyes. People were filing out of the auditorium. I thought I was finished, but then I was approached by a woman who I sensed had just entered the auditorium. She looked familiar, but I couldn't place her. Her smile jogged my memory. It was Shelly. I had not seen her in several years. She looked different—more beautiful and more at ease than when I'd last seen her, about five years earlier.

Just before she approached, I'd been packing my things, getting ready to leave. I was tired and looking forward to flying home, but something about her made me pause. She asked if she could share something with me. I hesitated for an instant; then our eyes met and I stopped what I was doing.

"You know," she started, "I've been through a lot since you last saw me—a lot. It's not important what happened, but I had a year . . . how can I describe it? You've heard of the dark night of the soul—mine lasted more than a year. I am not kidding." I could tell she wasn't. I suddenly recalled having heard a few years earlier from a student who was a close friend of hers that Shelly's intimate relationship of nearly ten years had ended and that, as a single mom, she had been struggling financially and emotionally.

"For much of it, I wasn't sure I was going to survive. I was in such a dark place. Many times I thought of three close relatives of mine who had committed suicide, and as hard as it is to admit, there were times when I thought that was how I might wind up, too.

"I can't explain why, but at one point, after more than a year of that darkness, I remembered that I had a meditation CD of yours. I'd never listened to it before, but something made me put it on. I did the practice where you guide people into a light in the heart. I think it's called the Healing the Heart Meditation. I listened to it. Two days later, I realized that I felt a little better, and I felt like the practice had something to do with how I was feeling. So I did the practice that day too, and again the next. I kept doing it day after day. I used it for months. Gradually it pulled me out of where I was, and now, two years later, my life is better than ever.

"Later, when I began to feel stronger and more positive, I started therapy. I wanted to understand what had led me to the place I'd been in. I learned a lot, enough to truly believe I'll never go back.

"I came here to thank you. I wanted to tell you how much of a difference you made in my life, even from a distance. I really don't know if I'd still be here if . . ." Her voice trailed off.

In her eyes I saw all that she had been through and her gratitude to have survived it. It was a powerful and moving moment. I was humbled to hear all that she'd overcome and of the Healing the Heart Meditation's pivotal role in turning her life around.

I'd seen and heard many versions of meditation's lifesaving capacities, but as Shelly told me her story I couldn't help thinking that something akin to grace had also played a part in her transformation. How else to explain the extent of her healing via something as subtle as a meditation that leads you into the light in your heart? How could something that simple so profoundly affect both her and her destiny? In approaching me to offer her thanks, Shelly sought to credit the role my CD had played in her breakthrough, but the truth was that it had nothing to do with me personally; it had everything to do with what becomes available to us through contentment.

> . . . .
>
> *Contentment expands your sense of what is possible by allowing you to experience the part of you that is, by its nature, limitless.*
>
> . . . .

Contentment is a many-faceted gem. Shelly's and Deborah's stories illuminate contentment's capacity to alleviate suffering, awaken dormant abilities, and fuel independence and personal freedom. As we've seen, contentment can spontaneously enliven your most constructive qualities and inspire you in ways that you might never have conceived of. Contentment also nurtures your capacity to let go and to accept. In addition to these extraordinarily positive effects, contentment expands your sense of what is possible by allowing you to experience the part of you that is, by its nature, limitless.

There is another facet of contentment that until now I have not addressed directly but which is implicit in every success story I've shared with you in this book. The ancient teachings tell us that making the light of contentment an ever-stronger presence in your life automatically leads you to your very best life. By establishing you in peace, self-reliance, and increasing levels of fearlessness, contentment empowers you to think and act in ways that are informed by your higher Self.

CHAPTER 28

THE WHITE HORSE

One of the most compelling texts in the Vedic tradition is the *Shvetash-vatara Upanishad*. *Shveta* is the Sanskrit word for "white," *ashva* means "horse," and *tara* means "supreme, excellent, the highest or most choice." Thus *shvetashvatara* means "the white horse that leads you to excellence or to the most supreme place." The central message of this text is that in order to reach everlasting fulfillment, you need to follow your "white horse." According to this scripture, this is another way of saying you can be led to your supreme life only by following the light of your true Self or Spirit, the light that is the Essence of all things and the source of contentment.

The *Shvetashvatara Upanishad* begins with a simple premise: we are always being led by something. In other words, throughout our lives one factor or another is always influencing us, propelling us toward what we become from one moment to the next, and ultimately to our unique destiny. This factor is what we point to when we try to explain who we are and where we find ourselves in life. For example, you might point to specific psychological factors having influenced your thoughts and actions. Someone else might point to world events, astrological factors, the culture in which he or she was raised, or socioeconomic background. Indisputably, something is always influencing you, shaping what you think, what you do, and even the words you use from moment to moment. As we've seen, Steven (who wanted to be healthy but continued abusing drugs and alcohol), Denise (who wanted a long-term relationship with a man but wouldn't acknowledge her anger and bitterness toward men), and Claudia (who wanted to start a school for children with special needs but wouldn't confront her lack of self-worth and take a systematic approach to overcoming it) consistently made decisions that were in conflict with their desires. All of them had more than enough evidence to suggest that their actions, thoughts, and words were not helping them get any closer to the fulfillment they sought. Nonetheless, something was pulling them in a direction other than the one that would lead them to act in their own best interests. The result was that they were led to destinies that were filled with more struggle, not less.

Whether we know it or not, we are all being led by a proverbial "horse." There are many varieties of horses, however, and according to the *Shvetashvatara Upanishad,* only a "white horse" is capable of leading you to your best life. The scripture's message is to find *shvetashvatara*—your white horse—so that you will be led to supreme happiness.

This scripture tells us that this white horse is the light of Spirit, Soul, or Essence, and it tells us where and how we can find this white horse.

> Omnipresent, dwelling in the heart of every living creature . . . He is the inner Self of all, hidden like a little flame in the heart. Only by a stilled mind can He be known . . . He who teaches each living creature to attain perfection according to its own nature.

The white horse, then, dwells "in the heart of every living creature." It is something everyone has access to, something permanent and ever-present that teaches you how "to attain perfection," and you can access it with a still mind. Therein lies the enduring message of this text: cultivate contentment, because contentment alone reveals the Intelligence that will guide you to your best life.

Shelly's emergence from her dark night of the soul is a powerful and poignant example of what happens when you let go of all the other horses and allow your white horse to lead you. Caught in a long downward spiral of despair, out of desperation she turned to meditation, which led her to the flame in her heart. The effect of doing so led her in a new direction filled with opportunities for lasting happiness that previously she had been unable to see; it may even have saved her life.

It's worth noting that the practice that Shelly happened upon, the

Healing the Heart Meditation, the one that effected such a powerful and positive change in her life, focused specifically on her heart and on light, both of which, the scripture instructs us, mark the path to the white horse ("He is the inner Self of all, hidden like a little flame in the heart").

Again, the teaching of the *Shvetashvatara Upanishad* emphasizes how important it is for you to cultivate a tranquil mind. As you do, your mind becomes clearer and clearer and, in the process, more and more able to know its Source. The more you experience contentment, the more the light of contentment illuminates your pathway to fulfill your soul's destiny. Over time, contentment becomes a powerful guiding force. Regularly accessing contentment enables you to see and make the choices that will lead to lasting fulfillment. Contentment gradually creates internal adjustments. At the same time, it directs you

> . . . .
> *Contentment alone reveals the Intelligence that will guide you to your best life.*
> . . . .

to make the external adjustments needed to help fulfill your soul's desires.

In making such a strong case for contentment, I don't want to leave you with the impression that contentment alone can solve everything. Steven experienced a measure of contentment through his yoga on a regular basis, yet because he never made the adjustments to give up his addictions, he never achieved his desire to get well. The lesson is that you need both contentment *and* adjustment; if you don't follow contentment's lead to make internal and external adjustments, you won't achieve your best life.

The Wisdom to Know What You Need

Let's return to the question I posed as the centerpiece of this section: how can you know which of the many steps in *The Four Desires* is the most critical for you to work with after you've completed the entire process?

The Serenity Prayer, a source of inspiration and guidance for millions of people around the world, provides a clue: "Grant us the serenity to accept the things we cannot change, courage to change the things we can, and the wisdom to know the difference." The phrase I want to focus on is "the *wisdom* to know the difference." The best advice I can offer about which steps in the process will be most vital to work with after you finish this book is for you to consistently spend time in the realm where the "wisdom to know" is most readily discovered: silence. The more time you spend in this sacred abode, the more your Higher Self will provide you with the answers you seek.

Trust that Providence will provide you with all the guidance and wisdom you will need. Knowing that your answer is never far away, have the intention and confidence that this wisdom will be revealed. If you get stuck or feel troubled over not yet fulfilling your intention, seek higher counsel. Pose your question to the light of your Higher Self, and in the days or weeks that follow, your answer will come. Listen for inner guidance and watch for signs that through its inherent compassion and wisdom your white horse is leading you. Recognize that you are part of Infinite Intelligence and that Creation is always guiding you.

Anna's Story

Anna had a successful career as an actress. For years she had starring roles in a long string of Spanish-language soap operas. When she and I sat down for her consultation, however, Anna told me that she wanted to do more with her life—something that could really touch and serve people. She wanted to make a difference. Her wish was to find an effective way to share the very thing that had brought immeasurable benefit to her life—yoga. Anna's desire was to bring yoga to the Spanish-speaking community, which she saw as lacking access to resources related to integrative health. She had made up her mind to do something about it.

After her second yoga teacher training course with me, she created and began teaching classes she called Yoga en Español. Despite Anna being a celebrity in her community and, you might think, the perfect ambassador to introduce it to yoga, her classes attracted only a small number of students. Instead of being discouraged, Anna focused on how much the students who did attend her classes appreciated what she had to offer.

Anna didn't quit her day job. She was a vital source of financial support for her family (all the more so because her husband was having health problems at the time), for the family of her recently deceased brother, and for her mother, who was in a hospital in grave condition. Anna continued teaching yoga, but given the small number of students in her yoga classes, she decided that a better way to reach her community would be to produce a *Yoga en Español* DVD and television series.

Teaching, plotting how to create a DVD, and juggling all the other demands in her life was a lot. She was struggling with these challenges when the two of us sat down for her consultation. She was frustrated that she was making so little progress on her dream of making a positive difference with her new project, and she was even more distressed by her family issues.

I suggested that she practice Relax into Greatness and continue to meditate regularly to lead her through this difficult time. "Sometimes, Anna," I said, "the only thing to do is the hardest thing to do—and that is nothing." I mentioned a poem from the *Zenrin Kushu*, a fifteenth-century anthology of Zen, Taoist, and Buddhist teachings:

> Sitting quietly, doing nothing,
> Spring comes, and the grass grows by itself.

I told Anna that contentment would allow her to embody patience and acceptance, and I suggested that she access contentment as consistently as possible. "Find a place of rest and tranquility, even in the midst of everything you have pulling at you right now," I suggested. "Never venture too far from it. It will be of immeasurable value. Trust that the seasons will change. Your spring will come, and the less you get caught up in the fact that it is not yet spring, the better your life will be."

I could tell by Anna's expression that what I'd said made sense to her, but I also knew that words alone were not going to relieve her of the anxiety and despair she felt. As I'd told her, sometimes doing nothing may be our best and only solution, but it isn't easily embraced, especially in difficult times.

> . . . .
> *Recognize that you are part of Infinite Intelligence and that Creation is always guiding you.*
> . . . .

Anna returned home and, hard as it was, made the time to practice Relax into Greatness and to meditate. She longed for things to be different, but instead of dwelling on her frustrations she found the strength to continue her commitments to practice and to work and not get bogged down in the challenges that were standing in the way of her dream. She was able to do this because she practiced abiding in contentment. Her daily meditation practice and regular relaxation sessions allowed her to access and continue to be led by her white horse.

For two years, Anna worked her day job as an actress, supported her family, and kept teaching yoga. In the meantime, without really thinking about how it was contributing to her goal, she was honing her skills and maturity as a teacher and refining ideas for a yoga DVD and television series. At one point during that second year, she took a few days to attend the Yoga of Fulfillment, and crafted a *sankalpa*. Seven months later, she sent me the following e-mail:

Dear Rod,

This is a quick note to share with you how wonderfully everything has turned out. I left the *Four Desires* seminar with the *sankalpa* "I'm in the perfect moment of my life to create, develop, and sell my DVD *Yoga en Español*" (as you know, I have been working on it for some time now).

For a long time I had planned to take a trip abroad with some dear friends. I had been so looking forward to it, pretty much counting on it as my reward for what has been a really difficult couple of years. But as the date to leave approached, my husband's health was still an issue, so I made the difficult decision not to go (I needed to be near him, not halfway around the world for a whole month). I felt sad and somewhat angry, but I came to accept it and did what I knew I had to do. I stayed home. Shortly afterward I decided I would use the time the best I could, which meant working on my *sankalpa* and everything else that needed taking care of.

Then, at the very time I had planned to be out of the country, I received a phone call from PBS. They were in the process of developing a network *en español* and were interested in developing a yoga show. The president of the network, it turns out, is a yoga practitioner and has had a dream to bring yoga to the Hispanic community.

They asked me to do a short routine, tape one of my classes, and do an interview on camera. They never used the word *casting*, saying only that they would be in touch if they decided to go forward with the project.

Three days later they called a meeting. When I got there I realized that they had cast several people throughout the United States to do the show. It was the producer's intention to have the show be led by a very fit and beautiful thirty-five-year-old woman. However, the board of directors at PBS, after seeing my interview, chose me (definitely older than thirty-five and closer to full-bodied than to very fit) to be the host of the show. They plan on producing the show and subsequent videos that will be distributed in the United States and Latin America. We start shooting on Monday. I've practically produced the show and designed the routines. They've put complete faith in me to create and lead the project.

I am very, very happy that finally my community will have *Yoga en Español* and that it will be available throughout the United States. I will be combining my two passions (yoga and TV). Yes, my *sankalpa* worked!

I wanted to share this with you, and thank you for your inspiration, teachings, support, and encouragement. A great part of this I owe to you.

Anna realized her dream. It was no accident. Like Karen, who found the perfect community and home for her family, Anna remained in the endeavor until she got there. She practiced all the steps in *The Four Desires,* but none was more important than addressing her need for *moksha,* cultivating her brightness during a time in her life that was otherwise less than light-filled.

The fact that Anna was able to find this vital support is a reminder of how contentment allows you to ride your "white horse" and let it lead you during even the most challenging times. Contentment does this by making it easier for you to practice *vairagya,* non-attachment, which means being able to let go and accept. For two years, Anna was able to authentically hold on to a measure of contentment despite the difficult challenges of her daily life. Even though it wasn't obvious to her when she was in the midst of it, contentment was pivotal to helping her be in the right place at the right time—and with the right attitude—to achieve her goal. Contentment was both Anna's solace in disquieting times and a powerful guide that throughout this period was giving shape and substance to the fulfillment of her dream.

Nurture Your Light

Thanks to maintaining her connection with her white horse, Anna was able to avoid something else that we are often prone to and that undermines us: the tendency to focus on what is *not* going well. It is easy to lose sight of all the things you have accomplished, the many blessings in your life, and even how far you have progressed toward your short- and long-term goals and instead obsess about what you see as the one thing in your life at which you are failing. Most of us are subject to this weakness—but your white horse is not.

Anna chose to nurture the light that is her white horse. By consistently returning to the light within her heart, by consistently dwelling in contentment, she managed to increase her appreciation for the gifts in her life and all that she had accomplished instead of dwelling on what she lacked or what was not going her way.

Anna's story reminds us once again that contentment is the eternal fountainhead that nurtures and feeds all the steps in *The Four Desires.* This is why, as we near the end of this book, I urge you to make time for it. In addition to all that I've written about it, contentment is also the key that unlocks the door to fulfilling your soul's desire for true freedom, the fourth desire or *moksha.* Without contentment, you are incapable of satisfying your longing to know something that truly endures, something that is limitless, eternal. Contentment is the ultimate (and only) means for your soul to see itself and thus for you to be reminded of just how blessed you are and always will be.

This particular facet of contentment frees you and allows you to step back and consider whether you are moving closer to or further away from your life's aim and purpose, your individual *dharma.* Abiding in contentment, you can clearly discern which of your past or future achievements has led or will lead you to fulfilling the deeper meaning and purpose of your life.

Deborah, who grew out of her habit of finding frustration and came to appreciate her already rich life, Shelly, who emerged from her dark night of the soul and found her joy again, and Anna, who fulfilled her dream of bringing yoga to a large Spanish-speaking community, all experienced the triumph of fulfillment through their work with contentment.

Establishing Your Practice

It's worth taking a final look at how the process of meditation can and does change your life, then identifying the steps of a regular meditation practice. Those of you who are new to meditation can use these steps to start meditating and to establish a regular practice. For both new and experienced meditators, this list of steps provides a useful framework to reflect on your experience of meditation.

A regular meditation practice progressively leads you through the following six steps:

1. Resolution
2. Practice
3. Attention
4. Self-awareness
5. Reprioritization
6. Adjustment

The first step to developing a meditation practice is resolving to practice, to make meditation a regular part of your life. This means organizing yourself and your life so that you have the space and time to do a practice. Do what you can. Even ten minutes a day can make a huge difference in the quality of your life. Once you've made your resolve, do the practice. Your practice must be consistent for an extended period of time. Keep in mind that it is better to do ten minutes a day every day than to do an hour once a week. Your practice should also be a meditation that you can embrace with at least some measure of enthusiasm or love. When first starting to meditate, you may find yourself resistant and critical of yourself for not doing it "better." Stick with it; overcome your resistance and self-criticism. Remember, doing even a short practice of, say, five to ten minutes, as long as it is done consistently, will gradually propel you toward the fruits of stillness.

Through consistent practice, your mind becomes more skilled at getting still; gradually it becomes able to turn inward and to perceive that you are more than just your body, more than just your thoughts. Over time, as you learn to settle and still your mind on a regular basis, you become more able to see your most positive qualities as well as your mind's self-defeating patterns and ideas. This pivotal step of the mind turning inward leads to greater self-awareness and to the discovery of what you are and what you are not.

Very often it's at this stage that more deep-seated forms of resistance will begin to surface. This may be a time when you will have to renew your resolve to continue. At this stage, you stand at the precipice of real and meaningful change and healing. As self-awareness grows, it naturally leads you to new understanding. You see with far greater clarity the deeper meaning and purpose of your life; you understand more about yourself, your needs, and your desires. Along with this awareness comes the recognition that true freedom or *moksha* is your key to lasting happiness and prosperity.

Increased self-awareness also helps you see the causes of your suffering and its underlying cures. This heightened perception brings with it an even greater level of contentment. It is at this point that you are often led to reconsider some of your basic assumptions about how best to live and about the things you want. You reprioritize. You let go of things that are no longer serving you, and you are more willing to embrace and move toward the things that do serve you. It's then that adjustment flows naturally, as your inner wisdom and the light of contentment guide you to make the internal and external changes that will lead you to who and what you are meant to be.

CHAPTER 29

YOUR SACRED JOURNEY

Paramahansa Yogananda once wrote, "It is better to die struggling than to abandon your efforts while there is still a possibility of accomplishing something more. . . . Analyze what you are, what you wish to become, and what shortcomings are impeding you. Decide the nature of your true task—your mission in life. Endeavor to make yourself what you should be and what you want to be."

You change your future by changing yourself. The more you insist on improving who and what you are, the more you become master of your destiny. Yet even when you've done everything you can, there will be times when you'll have little or nothing to show for your efforts. No matter, says the Bhagavad Gita, as long as you remember that fulfilling your *dharma*—the drive to become who and what you are meant to be—is the defining desire, the one that informs and gives shape to all others. "On this path [committed to *dharma*]," the Gita tells us, "effort never goes to waste, and there is no failure. . . . Perform work in this world . . . as a person established within himself—without selfish attachments, and alike in success and defeat."

Yogananda's words also serve as a reminder that there is no end to the process of fulfilling your destiny. You need only remain rightly committed to and focused on "your true task—your mission in life" and "what you should be and what you want to be."

Your soul or essence quietly watches. It never changes. It is the same now as it was when you were born, when you sat at your desk in grade school, when you first felt moved to help another person, when you first fell in love, when you first began to wonder about your place in the universe and how you would fulfill it. All the while your soul has retained its intrinsic connection to Creation, fully aware that life is the grandest and most sacred of all journeys and worthy of every effort to celebrate it.

The soul's timeless and luminous wisdom and compassion are always ready to lead you by means of the silent pull of desire. The more you are attuned to your soul, the more easily it can lead you to a fulfillment far beyond what most of us imagine is possible. That place is the fulfillment of *dharma,* the convergence of fate and destiny—a destination that awaits us and which can only be reached through the sum of all of our efforts.

> . . . .
>
> *The more you insist on improving who and what you are, the more you become master of your destiny.*
>
> . . . .

Dharma is Nature's grand plan, a tapestry with no beginning and no end. It is also the Intelligence that inspires and guides us to fulfill that plan. Responding to *dharma* is how you rise to become your most "mighty self." The *Pratyabhijnahrdayam,* a sacred tantric text, reminds us of this when it states, "On attaining strength, one makes the universe one's own." This teaching tells you everything you need to know: accept that the inherent nature of the world is sacred, know that you are a part of it, then live with the conviction always to challenge, to quest to become something more and better. "A man must never be satisfied with what he possesses," the Jain monk Somadeva Suri instructed. "Fortune abandons the man who is content with what he has."

Be prepared to let each successive step in your life ennoble you with more capacity. Resolve to become stronger and to fulfill your highest calling. With this commitment to yourself—and with love and respect for the world and the rest of creation—you will inevitably fulfill the lasting promise of yoga and all other spiritual traditions.

Grow. Determine to let nothing stand in your way. Reap the greatest riches life has to offer. Resolve to share the gifts you receive, enriching more and more lives with all that you discover and achieve.

My wish is that you will endeavor to brighten this world with the gifts of all that you have come to know as truly worthwhile and enduring. In the process, you will successfully embody the final teaching from the *Rig Veda,* the most ancient of all the Vedic texts, whose final lines tell us of this promise:

> May we walk together, talk together, and understand each other. Like bright beings joined in right thinking, may we share our bounty with each other.

REFLECTIONS ON WARRIOR III POSE

· · · ·

Virabhadrasana III

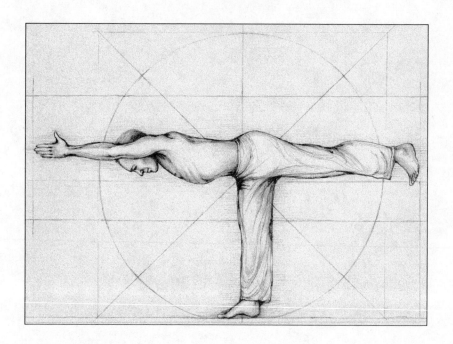

Warrior III is a standing balancing pose that challenges on many levels. The fact that Warrior III compels you to engage balance, flexibility, and stability simultaneously is one of the things that make it so formidable. Staying in the posture for as few as twenty seconds is a powerful exercise for the body and mind.

Unless you've practiced yoga, it's hard to know just how dynamic an endeavor it can be. It's surprising how something that appears so relatively static can also be demanding and intense. But *asana* is, and standing balancing postures such as Warrior III provide a particularly clear sense of this. They are also a perfect metaphor for the vital role that adjustment plays in allowing us to sustain fulfillment throughout the course of our lives.

From the moment you move into it, Warrior III gives you a lot of feedback. You might perceive the hamstring of your standing leg stretching, that your standing knee is unstable, that you are leaning too far to the left or right, that your breath is strained, or even that your heart is starting to race. The key to this pose—and every pose—is to stay aware enough while you are in it to constantly adjust to what you are experiencing.

The first step is to recognize that nothing in this world remains the same indefinitely. The ability to balance, for example, is less a static state than it is a momentary experience of equilibrium between two extremes. Being able to hold the pose means making constant microadjustments, responding to ever-changing conditions; doing so is the key to success. In the pose, this can mean adjusting your breath, relaxing or increasing your mental focus, stabilizing your standing leg, or making any one of dozens of other possible adjustments. In the context of life, adjustment refers to being aware and always being willing to respond to what life is trying to teach you.

From Now Till Forever

The following fable from the Vedic tradition serves as a beautiful reminder of something essential that is all too easily forgotten.

Many, many centuries ago, God was looking for a place to hide. You see, in those days She was receiving any and all who wanted to have an audience with Her. God's doors were open 24/7. All you had to do was knock on Her palace doors, wait your turn, and you would be received. It's no surprise that there was an endless line of devotees and seekers, as well as a lot of people who wanted stuff and who wanted to deliver their prayers directly to Her.

As was Her policy back then, God felt obliged to listen to each request. You can imagine that neither God, the angels, nor any of their attendants had a moment's rest. There were far too many people to attend to and too many requests to be heard. Some people were asking for their next child to be a girl; others were asking for a rich harvest, for it to rain or to stop raining, for more money, for healing for a sick relative, for help to see the future or to attain some extraordinary power, or that God would relieve them of grief and fear. It all got to be so much that God didn't have any time to attend to any godly business.

Having determined that something had to change, She convened all the greatest sages in order to discuss with them how to stem the constant flow of those looking to Her to fulfill all their desires and solve all their problems. The first sage suggested that they build Her a new palace at the highest point in the Himalayas, on Mount Everest. "No one has ever scaled Mount Everest," the sage said. "You will be undisturbed for eternity, and thus the natural order will be restored."

God shook Her head. "No," she said. "In a day or two [the ancient teachings tell us that a day in God's life is equivalent to a hundred thousand years in ours], human beings' desire and determination will allow them to get to the top of Everest. We'll need a different plan."

A second sage offered, "Let's build your new castle on the moon. Human beings will *never* get to the moon. There you will have all the quiet and peace you can imagine, and the order of things will be restored."

God just sighed and said, "No. In two or three days, human beings will find a way to get to the moon."

At a loss, all the sages fell silent.

"I have the answer," God said. "I'll put a small part of myself inside every person's heart. It will be the last place they'll look."

The clear moral of this fable is that a small piece of God is in every person's heart. Indeed, this is one of the paramount and most enduring messages of the Vedic tradition and, as I've said, the basis for being able to savor your work in the world while never becoming enslaved by it. Knowing the unconditional and boundless joy whose permanent abode is in your heart is the foundation for living your life with *moksha,* a true sense of freedom and fearlessness. This should remind all of us how enriching—in fact, invaluable—it is to learn to be in your heart. However, the tantric tradition provides us with another way of interpreting this fable.

> . . . .
>
> *Let the wisdom and love in your heart show you what and who you really are, then let it guide you.*
>
> . . . .

According to tantra, just below your heart center is something called the *ananda kanda*—the "root of bliss"—which is the source of the sublime contentment "enshrined" in or near your spiritual heart. If you are experiencing bliss, the teachings say, you are tapping into this root where your heart's blissful nature blossoms completely and endlessly. Within this root of bliss is the *kalpa vriksha,* the wishing tree. The teachings suggest that when you bring your desires with enough resolve to this tree, the tree then bestows on you the fulfillment of those desires.

How do you place your desires by your wishing tree with enough resolve? This book has been dedicated to answering that question. In many ways, answering it is its abiding message: Know that the world and everything in it, including you, is inherently sacred. Honor your place in it by respecting yourself and committing to becoming what you truly aspire to be. Understand that there is a truth that lies within you and can only be known by a still mind. Resolve to discover your Higher Self by looking inward. Once you glimpse this inner dimension—Essence, Source, Spirit—ask what desires *it* would have you fulfill. Set out in service of these desires and the greater good. Then, in full faith, take the loftiest of these desires back to your Source, which dwells in your heart, and let it lead you to them.

Let the wisdom and love in your heart show you what and who you really are, then let it guide you. Present your heart with a vision of what you know it longs for and it will help you fulfill the aspirations that have been in it all along. Make these steps your life's practice. In time, you will be richly rewarded and discover that for every step you have taken toward fulfilling your dreams, your dreams have taken a step toward you.

REFLECTIONS ON PERFECT SEAT POSE

· · · ·

Siddhasana

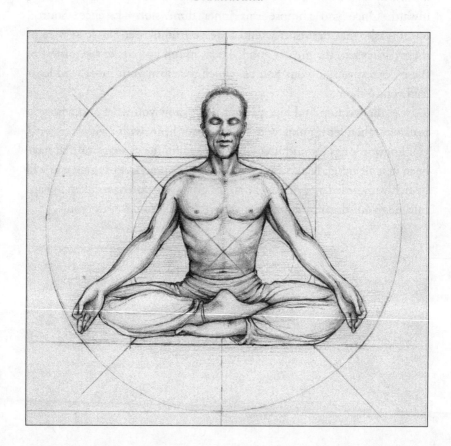

From the view of the ancient tradition, when yoga is practiced as a complete science, it allows us to embody the seven keys that open the door to spiritual and worldly fulfillment: purity, determination, steadiness, patience, lightness of the body, clear perception, and non-attachment. More than any other posture, Perfect Seat bestows these qualities.

Perfect Seat is the most important of all postures, according to the authoritative text *Hatha Yoga Pradipika*. Once this posture has been mastered, the text goes on to say, there is no need to practice any other. Given that the posture appears to be little more than sitting upright, the idea of it being the most important might seem counterintuitive. But break the pose down and you begin to recognize that sitting upright on the floor with your head, neck, and torso in a straight line involves many distinct actions. First, it requires flexibility in the hips, legs, ankles, and lower back. The ability to fully lift your chest and be free from tension in the neck and shoulders is also necessary. A surprising element that allows us to hold the pose comfortably is strength, particularly in the lower back and abdominal muscles. Consider all of these component parts and it becomes clearer why this may well be the most important of all postures. The simple fact is that in order to be able to access the depths of Perfect Seat, we need the conditioning that all of the other poses (forward bends, backbends, twists, lateral poses, extensions, and inversions) provide.

There is perhaps an even more compelling reason why this pose is considered so significant: because the posture doesn't involve any kind of deep stretch, the work it requires is mostly internal. Once you can sit in this posture comfortably, you measure mastery in it not by what you can do with your body, but by what you can do with your mind. This means that the pose becomes fully alive, fully realized, when you can rest in it and fully sense that you are the embodiment of everything to which you aspire.

Perfect Seat is the culmination of practice because it moves you beyond the physical aspect of "doing" *asana* and toward the experience that the body is a universe unto itself. When you become completely absorbed in Perfect Seat, the spine is extended and completely aligned, and you become steeped in a state of profound and effortless awareness. Fully absorbed in the pose, you sense that there is nowhere to go; there is no experience, no feeling that you desire that can't be found within.

. . . .

ACKNOWLEDGMENTS

I am blessed and privileged to have studied with two great masters. Their effect on me, both personally and professionally, has shaped my life in inestimable ways. All that I have amounted to as a teacher, and whatever personal advances I have made toward the promise of the sublime and timeless wisdom of the Vedic tradition, come from having been graced by their accomplishments, love, and generosity. Kavi Yogiraj Mani Finger was the first to lead me into the treasures of yoga and tantra, two of many systems to have come from the Vedas. My other great influence and current teacher is Pandit Rajmani Tigunait. It is thanks to his wisdom, erudition, and kind embrace of me as his student that my life today is as fulfilling as it is, and that this book exists.

Two significant things happened upon my meeting "Panditji." The first was the immediate realization that I had spent twenty years practicing, studying, and teaching yoga to prepare for all that he would reveal to me. The second was that it sparked a kind of fire, because in the weeks that followed, the first outline and much of the subject matter for this book began to unfold. The sheer force of his love of life and his brilliance in deciphering the ancient wisdom are, by far, the greatest influence on my life and on *The Four Desires*.

I would be remiss if I failed to acknowledge as well Sri Swami Rama. Although I never met or studied with him personally, his presence, teachings, writings, and the light of the wisdom he passed onto my teacher

Pandit Rajmani Tigunait are vital touchstones woven throughout the pages in this book.

When I have quoted Mani, Panditji, and Swami Rama directly, I have attributed it to them. However, so much of what I learned from them is woven into the ideas of *The Four Desires* that it is impossible for me to separate the strands that they contributed from the whole of the tapestry that is this book. I am eternally grateful to them as well as to Mani's son, Yogiraj Alan Finger, who was my initial link to the timeless succession of luminous teachers, masters, and sages who have lit a golden path to eternal fulfillment. There will never be words to adequately express the depth of my gratitude.

It took three different editors at Random House to bring *The Four Desires* to fruition. Each successive changing of the guard contributed a new vision and, in the end, helped to make this book what I hoped it would be. Each played a vital role in the significant task of publishing the book. First and foremost, I wish to acknowledge Toni Burbank, not just because she believed in the project enough to say yes. It was the prospect of collaborating with her, one of the most brilliant, insightful, and charming nonfiction editors in the contemporary publishing world, that made me choose Random House as my publisher. To Beth Rashbaum, who took the reins next, thank you for your enthusiasm, keen eye, and the key role you played in shaping the manuscript. And finally, thank you to Marnie Cochran, who, with her savvy and attention to detail, saw things that the rest of us didn't and gave the book its final form.

I must acknowledge Mark Bruce Rosin, who turned out to be the book's principal editorial patron. Shortly after we began working together, it was clear that Mark was a meticulous and exacting editor. But as the weeks of working together passed into months, Mark never failed to ensure that the teachings and the processes that I intended to walk the reader through were clearly presented on the page. I will always be indebted to his generosity and to his being an invaluable amalgam: editor, literary consultant, champion for *The Four Desires* and the ancient teachings it draws from, as well as dear friend.

Thank you, too, to the staff at ParaYoga's offices: to Sherry Karu for your grace and willingness to be with me every step of the way and to Berit Daniels for being so good at what you do.

Thanks as well to the following for their contributions to the book: Ben Felcher, Bijan Amini, Charlie, Claudette Araujo, Cynthia Hopenfeld Rosin, David Vigliano, the Dorazios, Doug Ellis, Fila Dominguez, Greg Lichtenberg, Jordan Roberts, Joshua Gross, Kate Ramirez, Kathy O'Rourke, Lauren Toolin, Lynn Mathews, Marion Gross, Michael Harriot, Moises Aavedra, Peggy Garrity, Dr. Stephen Stiteler, Sue Neufeld, and the Sullivans.

A final and heartfelt thanks to everyone who has participated in the Yoga of Fulfillment workshops over the years and particularly to those whose stories appear in these pages.

. . . .

NOTES

Introduction

xi "The wings of humankind is its aspiration" Jalalu'ddin Rumi, *The Illustrated Rumi: A Treasury of Wisdom from the Poet of the Soul* (HarperOne, 2000), 154.

xvi "Quiet desperation" Henry David Thoreau, *Walden* (Beacon Press, 2004), xv.

xxi "Follow that advice of mine" Pandit Rajmani Tigunait, *Seven Systems of Indian Philosophy* (Himalayan Institute Press, 1983), 7.

xxi "Deep within lies" Pandit Rajmani Tigunait, *From Death to Birth: Understanding Karma and Renunciation: The Wisdom of God* (Himalayan Institute Press, 1997), 44.

Chapter 1

5 "The species which has" Pandit Rajmani Tigunait, "Power and Privilege," *Yoga International,* no. 110, 2010, 51.

5 "The important thing is this" Marie-Anne Gouhier, *Charles Du Bos* (Simon & Schuster, 2008), 39 ("premier tressaillement vital; surtout il s'agit à tout moment de sacrifier ce que nous sommes à ce que nous pouvons devenir").

7 "Man is verily formed of desire" Arthur Avalon, *Mahanirvana Tantra* (Dover Publications, 1972), cxxxviii.

7 "As long as one has a body" Eknath Easwaran, *The Bhagavad Gita* (Nilgiri Press, 2007), 58.

8 The first step in yoga T. K. V. Desikachar, *Religiousness in Yoga: Lectures on Theory and Practice* (University Press of America, 1980), 42.

8 "On the physical" Alain Daniélou, *Virtue, Success, Pleasure, and Liberation: The Four Aims of Life in the Tradition of Ancient India* (Inner Traditions International, 1993), 111.

Chapter 2

10 "It is not inaccessible" Swami Venkatesananda, *The Concise Yoga Vasistha* (State University of New York Press, 1984), 43.

10 "Only by the stilled mind" Eknath Easwaran, *The Upanishads* (Nilgiri Press, 2007), 167.

11 "According to most" Pandit Rajmani Tigunait, *Tantra Unveiled* (Himalayan Institute Press), 1.

12 "The thirst for life" Arthur Avalon, *Mahanirvana Tantra* (Dover Publications, 1972), 90–91.

13 "All—whatsoever that moves in the universe" Swami Rama, *Living with the Himalayan Masters* (Himalayan Institute Press, 2007), 223.

13 "Desire is the essence of all" Alain Daniélou, *Virtue, Success, Pleasure, and Liberation: The Four Aims of Life in the Tradition of Ancient India* (Inner Traditions International, 1993), 110.

13 "Both renunciation of action" Eknath Easwaran, *The Bhagavad Gita* (Nilgiri Press, 2007), 127.

13 "Desire is not to be let" Arthur Avalon, *Mahanirvana Tantra* (Dover Publications, 1972), 91.

15 "What is here is elsewhere" Arthur Avalon, *Mahanirvana Tantra* (Dover Publications, 1972), 28.

15 "Tantric masters discovered long ago" Pandit Rajmani Tigunait, *Tantra Unveiled* (Himalayan Institute Press, 2007), 2.

Chapter 3

18 "Omnipresent, dwelling in the heart" Eknath Easwaran, *The Upanishads* (Nilgiri Press, 2007), 167.

20 "That course of meritorious action" Arthur Avalon, *Mahanirvana Tantra* (Dover Publications, 1972), 91.

22 "He who does not desire pleasure" Alain Daniélou, *Virtue, Success, Pleasure, and Liberation: The Four Aims of Life in the Tradition of Ancient India* (Inner Traditions International, 1993), 110.

22 "The merchant, the laborer, the gods" Alain Daniélou, *Virtue, Success, Pleasure, and Liberation: The Four Aims of Life in the Tradition of Ancient India* (Inner Traditions International, 1993), 111.

CHAPTER 4

29 "Fetal cells destined" Linda Acredolo and Susan Goodwyn, *Baby Minds: Brain-Building Games Your Baby Will Love* (Bantam, 2000), 2–4.

31 "All matter originates and exists" Gregg Braden, *The Divine Matrix: Bridging Time, Space, Miracles, and Belief* (Hay House, 2008), vii.

31 "The eternal and immutable principles" Arthur Avalon, *Mahanirvana Tantra* (Dover Publications, 1972), 91.

32 A human being is part John Borysenko and Larry Rothstein, *Minding the Body, Mending the Mind* (Bantam, 1988), 103.

CHAPTER 5

38 "It is better to perform" Eknath Easwaran, *The Bhagavad Gita* (Nilgiri Press, 2007), 262.

38 "This is the true joy in life" George Bernard Shaw, *Man and Superman* (IndoEuropeanPublishing.com, 2010), 18.

38 "The masterpiece of man, is to" Benjamin Franklin, *Poor Richard's Almanack* (Barnes & Noble Books, 2004), 48.

38 "Analyze what you are" Paramahansa Yogananda, *The Law of Success: Using the Power of Spirit to Create Health, Prosperity, and Happiness* (Self-Realization Fellowship, 1989), 16.

45 "You are what your deep, driving" Eknath Easwaran, *The Upanishads* (Nilgiri Press, 2007), 33.

CHAPTER 6

47 "I want to be useful" Anne Frank, *The Diary of a Young Girl* (Everyman's Library, 2010), 251.

51 "There will never be" Swami Satyananda Saraswati, *High On Waves* (Yoga Publications Trust, first edition 2009).

Chapter 8

80 **"Once you make a decision"** Ichak Adizes, *Mastering Change: The Power of Mutual Trust and Respect* (Adizes Institute Publishing, 1992), 229.

80 **"If you cling to a certain"** Paramahansa Yogananda, *The Law of Success: Using the Power of Spirit to Create Health, Prosperity, and Happiness* (Self-Realization Fellowship, 1989), 9.

81 **"Four out of five people"** Tara Parker-Pope, "Will Your Resolutions Last Until February?" *New York Times,* December 31, 2007.

82 **"On this path you must"** Pandit Rajmani Tigunait, *At the Eleventh Hour: The Biography of Swami Rama* (Himalayan Institute Press, 2001), 316.

82 **"The mind is everything"** Sir John Templeton, *Wisdom from World Religions: Pathways Toward Heaven on Earth* (Templeton Foundation Press, 2002), 1.

85 **"For those who lack resolution"** Eknath Easwaran, *The Bhagavad Gita* (Nilgiri Press, 2007), 93.

86 **"Researchers at Columbia University"** Jim Holt, "The Year in Ideas: A to Z; Prayer Works," *New York Times,* December 9, 2001.

Chapter 9

90 **"His desires are right desires"** Swami Prabhavananda and Frederick Manchester, *The Upanishads: Breath from the Eternal* (New American Library, 2002), 74.

90 **"I am desire itself"** Eknath Easwaran, *The Bhagavad Gita* (Nilgiri Press, 2007), 153.

90 **"This self is neither far"** Swami Venkatesananda, *The Concise Yoga Vasistha* (State University of New York Press, 1984), 43.

Chapter 11

118 **"Man proposes, God disposes"** Ludovico Ariosto, *Orlando Furioso* (Oxford University Press, 2008), 561.

Chapter 12

128 **Bengali Baba** Pandit Rajmani Tigunait, *At the Eleventh Hour: The Biography of Swami Rama* (Himalayan Institute Press, 2001), 58.

129 **"Strengthen your mind"** Paramahansa Yogananda, *The Law of Success: Using the Power of Spirit to Create Health, Prosperity, and Happiness* (Self-Realization Fellowship, 1989), 31.

CHAPTER 13

140 **"You are what your deep, driving"** Eknath Easwaran, *The Upanishads* (Nilgiri Press, 2007), 33.

144 **"If you want to identify"** Thomas Merton, *My Argument with the Gestapo* (New Directions, 1975), 160.

CHAPTER 14

158 **"People undergoing radical"** Larry Dossey, *Healing Words* (Harper-Collins), 64.

161 **"Regions of the brain associated"** Natalie Angier, "Brain Is a Co-Conspirator in a Vicious Stress Loop," *New York Times,* August 17, 2009.

CHAPTER 15

174 **"Success is hastened or delayed"** Paramahansa Yogananda, *The Law of Success: Using the Power of Spirit to Create Health, Prosperity, and Happiness* (Self-Realization Fellowship, 1989), 20.

CHAPTER 16

187 **"Creation is only the projection"** Swami Prabhavananda, *Srimad Bhagavatam: The Wisdom of God* (Capricorn Books, 1968), 37.

CHAPTER 17

197 **"God's plan for us often"** Paramahansa Yogananda, *The Law of Success: Using the Power of Spirit to Create Health, Prosperity, and Happiness* (Self-Realization Fellowship, 1989), 24.

198 **"By mastering *samyama*"** Swami Satyananda Saraswati, *Four Chapters on Freedom: Commentary on the Yoga Sutras of Patanjali* (Yoga Publications Trust, 2002), 232.

199 **"I trust my gut"** Karen Salmansohn, *Gut: How to Think from Your Middle to Get to the Top* (HOW Books, 2006), 34.

199 **"My funny bone instinct kept urging me"** Craig Karges, *Ignite Your Intuition* (Health Communications, 1999), 39.

199 **"I know when I have a problem"** Craig Karges, *Ignite Your Intuition* (Health Communications, 1999), 42.

200 **"When you develop true sensitivity"** Swami Satyananda Saraswati, *A Systematic Course in the Ancient Tantric Techniques of Yoga and Kriya* (Bihar School of Yoga, 1981), 601.

Chapter 20

234 **"Yoga is the breaking of contact with pain"** Swami Prabhavananda and Christopher Isherwood, *Bhagavad Gita* (Signet Classic, 2002), 66.

234 **"Seek refuge in the attitude"** Eknath Easwaran, *Bhagavad Gita* (Nilgiri Press, 2007), 94.

235 **"The awakened sages call a person"** Eknath Easwaran, *Bhagavad Gita* (Nilgiri Press, 2007), 118.

Chapter 21

242 **"Wise, ever satisfied"** Eknath Easwaran, *Bhagavad Gita* (Nilgiri Press, 2007), 118.

247 **"Reshape yourself through"** Eknath Easwaran, *Bhagavad Gita* (Nilgiri Press, 2007), 47.

Chapter 22

250 **"The important thing is this"** Marie Anne Gouhier, *Charles Du Bos* (Simon & Schuster, 2008), 39 ("premier tressaillement vital; surtout il s'agit à tout moment de sacrifier ce que nous sommes à ce que nous pouvons devenir").

Chapter 23

255 **"Self-preservation or attachment"** Swami Satyananda Saraswati, *Four Chapters on Freedom: Commentary on the Yoga Sutras of Patanjali* (Yoga Publications Trust, 2002), 2–9.

257 **"The fire of knowledge"** Eknath Easwaran, *Bhagavad Gita* (Nilgiri Press, 2007), 119.

257 **"Of the four aims"** Arthur Avalon, *Mahanirvana Tantra* (Dover Publications, 2009), 86.

257 **"The Self cannot be pierced"** Eknath Easwaran, *Bhagavad Gita* (Nilgiri Press, 2007), 91.

Chapter 24

270 **"The sustained effort"** Swami Satyananda Saraswati, *Four Chapters on Freedom: Commentary on the Yoga Sutras of Patanjali* (Yoga Publications Trust, 2002), 59.

CHAPTER 26

284 **"The tendency to avoid is stronger"** Charles L. Scott, *Handbook of Correctional Mental Health* (American Psychiatric Publishing, 2009), 202.

CHAPTER 27

293 **"This self is neither far"** Swami Venkatesananda, *The Concise Yoga Vasistha* (State University of New York Press, 1984), 43.

CHAPTER 28

298 **"Omnipresent, dwelling in the heart"** Eknath Easwaran, *The Upanishads* (Nilgiri Press, 2007), 167.
299 **"Grant us the serenity"** AA Services, *The Big Book, 4th edition* (Alcoholics Anonymous World Services, Inc., 2001), 357.
301 **"Sitting quietly, doing nothing"** From the *Zenrin Kushu,* cited in Alan Watts, *The Way of Zen* (Vintage, 1999), 134.

CHAPTER 29

307 **"It is better to die struggling"** Paramahansa Yogananda, *The Law of Success: Using the Power of Spirit to Create Health, Prosperity, and Happiness* (Self-Realization Fellowship, 1989), 14.
307 **"On this path"** Eknath Easwaran, *The End of Sorrow: The Bhagavad Gita for Daily Living* (Nilgiri Press, 1993), 89, 98.
308 **"On attaining strength"** Swami Shantananda and Peggy Bendet, *The Splendor of Recognition* (SYDA Foundation, 2003), 283.
308 **"A man must never"** Alain Daniélou, *Virtue, Success, Pleasure, and Liberation: The Four Aims of Life in the Tradition of Ancient India* (Inner Traditions International, 1993), 101.
309 **"May we walk together"** Pandit Rajmani Tigunait, *Lighting the Flame of Compassion* (Himalayan Institute Press, 2004), 7.

Rod Stryker is widely considered one of the preeminent yoga, tantra, and meditation teachers in the United States. He is renowned for his depth of knowledge, practical wisdom, and unique ability to transmit the deepest aspects of these teachings and practices to modern audiences and students from all walks of life. Rod is the founder of Para Yoga® and has taught for more than thirty years, training teachers and leading seminars, retreats, and workshops throughout the world.

Stryker began his intensive study and practice of yoga at age nineteen. Two years later, he began a nearly two-decade-long apprenticeship with internationally renowned yoga master Kavi Yogiraj Mani Finger and his son, Yogiraj Alan Finger. Eventually, he would become his teachers' only American disciple to be given the title Yogiraj, master of Yoga. Rod met his current teacher, Pandit Rajmani Tigunait, Ph.D., spiritual head of the Himalayan Institute, in 1999.

Acclaimed as a leading voice for the ancient traditions, accomplished yogi, teacher, lecturer, and writer, Rod has a down-to-earth approach informed as much by his mastery of the sublime teachings as by his love of life and devotion to his wife and four children. He lives with his family in Colorado.